Reflections on Freedom

Daily Meditations
On The Steps Of Recovery

Written by Members of
Nicotine Anonymous (NicA)

Dallas, Texas

First Edition 2021

ISBN: 978-1-7338939-5-4

Published by Nicotine Anonymous World Services,
a non-profit tax-exempt corporation.

Printed in the United States

Nicotine Anonymous website address:
www.nicotine-anonymous.org

Preface

The experience, strength, and hope in these writings came from the individual contributions of Nicotine Anonymous (NicA) members. Trusted servants, appointed by the chairperson of Nicotine Anonymous World Services, collected, edited, arranged, and formatted these writings as 366 daily meditations for publication. In response to a number of members' requests, each of the twelve months contains several meditations that correspond, by the month's number, to each one of the Twelve Steps of Nicotine Anonymous. For example, January contains several meditations related to Step One, February to Step Two, and so on throughout the book. An index is provided in the back of the book so that members can also search by topic. In 2021, the World Services Conference delegates voted to approve the content.

We express our gratitude to all who contributed toward our fellowship's primary purpose to carry the Nicotine Anonymous message of recovery to any nicotine addict who still suffers. May this book help all members to find the peace that we seek, and to practice the principles in all our affairs.

Our Preamble

Nicotine Anonymous is a fellowship of people helping each other to live our lives free of nicotine. We share our experience, strength, and hope with each other so that we may be free from this powerful addiction. The only requirement for membership is the desire to stop using nicotine. There are no dues or fees for Nicotine Anonymous membership; we are self-supporting through our own contributions. Nicotine Anonymous is not allied with any sect, denomination, political entity, organization or institution, does not engage in any controversy, neither endorses nor opposes any cause. Our primary purpose is to offer support to those who are trying to gain freedom from nicotin

REPRINTED AND ADAPTED WITH PERMISSION OF THE AA. GRAPVINE

Excerpts From Our Literature

***Nicotine Anonymous: The Book,* section Step Eleven**

"[Meditation] helps us go inside ourselves, to be quiet, and to empty ourselves so our Higher Power can come in and fill us up."

"Serenity Prayer for Nicotine Users" *(pamphlet)*

"Remember, it is not really the stress, frustration or even the craving that causes us to keep using nicotine again, but rather our lack of serenity and courage to deal with the craving."

"Our Policy of Openness: Our Higher Power As We May Each Come to Understand" *(pamphlet)*

"Nicotine Anonymous is not a religion, nor does it have an "official" or "approved" spiritual path. Our program is based on universal spiritual principles and uses the concept referred to as God, Higher Power, or a Power greater than ourselves as an essential means to recover from our active nicotine addiction."

"Slogans To Help Us Be Happy, Joyous and Free Living Without Nicotine" *(pamphlet)*

Look for the Lesson

If we consider accepting the events of our day as lessons, we can learn. An open mind receives. The lessons delivered to us today may be about either acceptance, courage, humility, compassion or whatever issues we need to work on.

Our Three Conference-Approved Prayers

The Serenity Prayer

God, grant me serenity to accept the things I cannot change, courage to change the things I can, and wisdom to know the difference.

—Selected from text written by Reinhold Niebuhr, 1926

Third Step Prayer

Relieve me of the bondage of self.
Help me abandon myself to the spirit.

Move me to do good in this world and show kindness.
Help me to overcome and avoid anger, resentment, jealousy,
and any other kind of negative thinking today.

Help me to help those who suffer.
Keep me alert with courage to face life and not withdraw from it,
not to insulate myself from all pain whereby I insulate myself
from love as well.

Free me from fantasy and fear. Inspire and direct
my thinking today; let it be divorced from self-pity,
dishonesty and self-seeking motives.

Show me the way of patience, tolerance, kindliness, and love.

I pray for all of those to whom I've been unkind and ask that they
are granted the same peace that I seek.

Seventh Step Prayer

My Higher Power, I place myself in your hands and humbly ask
that my character defects be lifted from me so that I may help
others. Please grant me willingness, courage, and strength so
that through my actions I may reflect your love and wisdom. Amen.

JANUARY 1

We took a realistic look at the power nicotine had over
us and we saw that its control was absolute.
—*Nicotine Anonymous: The Book*

With Step One, I admitted I was powerless over nicotine. Then came the awareness of how powerless I was. And the more I attended meetings, the more I came face to face with the fact that I could not control my craving for nicotine.

Attending meetings totally wrecked my smoking. I no longer enjoyed, but hated smoking. Clearly smoking was robbing me of my life. As I continued to show up at meetings, the agony of my unrelenting addiction continued. I straddled that fence of appeasing the cravings and hating myself for giving in.

It appeared the only way out was to go through it, face the cravings and whatever came next. I had the unconditional love and support of the God of my understanding, my fellow nicotine addicts, and my sponsor. They understood what I was going through.

More than anything I wanted to feel good again, have a better quality of life, and to shed the unrelenting power of nicotine. Admitting my powerlessness over nicotine was the first step to this amazing and beautiful life in recovery.

Today, dear Higher Power, help me see past the end of my nose and proactively plan for a better quality of life.

JANUARY 2

Just as soon as we make a good resolution,
we get into a situation
which makes its observance unbearable.
—William Feather

I have made numerous New Year's resolutions to stop using nicotine. I announced my intentions to family and friends as an incentive. I have bet money or asked for a financial reward to keep my focus on gaining benefits. However, whatever resoluteness I began with dissolved shortly afterwards.

Even if I endured the physical cravings, stressful emotional or psychologically challenging situations would wear me down until I felt life was unbearable. I had to admit that asking myself to stop a physical and mental disease with just words, sincere as they were, was not manageable on my own.

I joined an online Nicotine Anonymous meeting. The connection with others who understood what I was going through was uplifting. As I worked the Steps, I came to believe that this addiction has a spiritual solution. Allowing my Higher Power's and others' support and acceptance has its own rewards and benefits. I belong, and I have a lot to look forward to.

---

*Today, I manage my daily challenges, because I have
the guidance of a recovery program,
the care of a power greater than myself,
and the understanding of my fellow members.*

JANUARY 3

Every moment is a chance of a lifetime.
—Pir Vilayat Inayat Khan

Beginnings are dynamic moments. A beginning happens in the moment between letting go and reaching forward. It is where I cast my net of hope. I wonder if I will catch the expected or unexpected? I won't know until I begin.

Sadly, many beginnings I could have had were stalled for years. As a nicotine addict, I admit that letting go of the familiar, facing the unknown was especially difficult for me. Start a day without smoking? How could I cope without nicotine? I couldn't tolerate the discomfort of a craving for a few minutes. I justified my excuses to placate my failures, and shrouded myself in denial to hide fear. But when nothing changed, nothing changed.

With recovery, I accept that beginnings wait within me, longing to emerge into the sunlight of the spirit. The combined hope of the NicA fellowship's members inspires me to see that I have beginnings beyond my present, limited beliefs.

Meetings offer me real examples of progress through members' experience, strength, and hope. Our program of recovery continually offers opportunities for spiritual growth. I must take the chance to change within this lifetime.

Today, I am willing to begin the next step in my recovery and answer the opportunity that is knocking before me.

JANUARY 4

Step One was not an intellectual exercise.

—Nicotine Anonymous: The Book

Before finding NicA, I had wanted to get free of this madness, this nicotine trap, for years. Although I was good with my hands and quite adept at using my brain at problem solving, I just couldn't figure my way out of nicotine's grip. Oh, I'd get ideas, then try to psych myself up, but I would always cave to the crave and return to the isolation of addiction.

This problem was not outside of me where I might see a way to deal with it. Addiction is invisible, and it was inside me. The smoke may have appeared as a screen or buffer against my outer world, yet its effect separated me from my inner self as well. I wanted to get free, but in awkward or challenging moments, the addiction would have me withdraw rather than face the withdrawal. No matter how I appeared to others, I was isolated in my cave.

Joining NicA gave me a higher intervention, a Higher Inspiration. With each meeting, I ventured further out from the cave. Because my intellectual musings and problem-solving routines were not enough to restore me to sanity, when I combined them with the power of positive belief, the spiritual awakening process lifted me free from the addiction.

Today, I improve my conscious contact
with my Higher Inspiration.

JANUARY 5

A thing that has not been begun cannot be finished.
—Robert Henri

Start. Start something I want. Start something I dream of doing. Lean forward and start. To start is to summon the power of nature that desires its fulfillment.

I may not know at first whether I will finish or be successful, but the opportunity for completion only happens as a result of beginning. Step One was a beginning. It may take numerous attempts to achieve. As with exercise, I can become continually stronger with repeated effort.

When I started living nicotine free, so much became possible. My strength and my senses returned. Now whatever I start, there's a better chance I'll finish.

Addiction trapped me for years. Recovery helps me to begin what I dream of doing. Once I experience movement, it builds momentum. This action creates hope. I receive the joys of finishing, because I've found the support to start.

Today, I am at the starting line of my life,
and I receive the joys of achieving my dreams.

JANUARY 6

We are more disturbed by a calamity which threatens us
than by one which has befallen us.
—John Lancaster Spalding

How many moments did I spend agonizing about even the prospect of living without nicotine? Stop using nicotine forever? Just the thought of being deprived, even temporarily, would most certainly cause the urgency to use my drug of choice.

Those who have never felt the anxiety of impending physical and psychological deprivation from nicotine cannot understand. With all the friendly cartoons, smiling faces, and catchy slogans, I should not have been mystified as to how something which was made to appear so nice could have such a monstrous power over me.

For me, the actual withdrawal from nicotine was difficult, yet it was less difficult than I had imagined with such dread. Nicotine addiction is a mental, physical, and spiritual disease. I can ease the big panic if I remember to keep it simple and reach out for help from my Higher Power, my sponsor, and my group. I am, just for today, using our five Tools of recovery: meetings, literature, service, group contact list and sponsorship. And I choose to pick up the Tools instead of another dose of nicotine.

Today, any fear I project is often worse
than the actual challenge that I face.

JANUARY 7

Just Keep Showing Up at meetings…until you like going!
—Nicotine Anonymous Member

As a newcomer I felt uncomfortable sitting in a room with strangers without using nicotine and admitting I had failed to quit on my own. After a few meetings, I saw that members offer understanding, not criticism. Still, hearing others talk about surrendering baffled me because I was trying to gain control, not give up control.

It was frightening when others were able to quit. The reality that I might actually be separated from my perceived best buddy was scary. I had a lot of mixed feelings during the meetings, and certainly had doubts that I could stay the course. But I knew my only alternative was to keep on smoking, and that was making my life downright unmanageable.

To feel comfortable at meetings, it took me showing up a number of times. I kept coming back and gradually felt more at ease, and made a decision that I would **Keep Showing Up** for my recovery. I began to feel and even believe there was hope for me. Once I accepted that my initial discomfort was worth the gift of receiving the support of my fellow members, I came to like meetings. Pushing through the discomfort, I found hope and understanding. I came to believe I could surrender with the help of my fellow nicotine addicts and a benevolent Higher Power.

Today, I accept that crossing a bridge of discomfort can bring me to a new place of joy.

JANUARY 8

We admitted we were powerless over nicotine—
that our lives had become unmanageable.
—Step One

As a nicotine addict, I had to become aware of the unmanageability of my life before I could admit my powerlessness. I was told by a medical professional that I needed to stop using nicotine, or in the next five years I would face serious health consequences. This wakeup call showed me the unmanageability that nicotine was causing in my life. My addiction had fooled me into thinking that I would escape the harmful effects of smoking, or that I could stop someday before my health deteriorated.

Deep down I knew that I was powerless over nicotine, because I had wanted to stop for a long time. But I never seemed to be able to overcome the powerful withdrawal pangs on my own. Usually, I would last until about 11 a.m. on a quit day before giving in and smoking.

I needed to reach out and ask for help from others. Nicotine Anonymous gave me that help and great hope for living nicotine free. By attending meetings, I am reaching out and asking for help from others. The more I open up and share my difficulties and my triumphs, and the more I listen to others at meetings, the more I understand myself and my addiction. I participate in my recovery one day at a time.

Today, I reach out for help from others,
and my life is becoming more manageable.

I didn't get to my bottom because I was so damn smart.

—Nicotine Anonymous Member

When I was a child, I watched my smart parents use nicotine. I listened as advertising told me how smart I would be to choose a certain brand. I didn't want to appear stupid. Once the adult messages were implanted in my young mind, my behavior was destined to follow. After I put the first few puffs into my body, nicotine was in control. Hey, I thought I knew what I was doing, but obviously I wasn't all that smart. Nicotine is powerful, yet subtle. When I used it, my brain was not clear on how the drug was affecting me. Nicotine hid its damage for years.

Nicotine is cunning. It outsmarted me even after I caught on to its effects. I didn't seek help until my body and spirit were screaming. I listened to the unrelenting voice in my head saying, "This is your life calling," until I finally reached out for help and found relief in Nicotine Anonymous.

I have stopped using nicotine, but I accept nicotine memories could tempt me again. My recovery has not been due to my intellect. Recovery happened by answering the call from my heart, and the result has been a spiritual awakening that guides me, each day, one day at a time.

Today, I manage my life using this program,
the smartest decision I ever made.

JANUARY 10

If I'm ever feeling down,
I just type "Yo are the best" into a search engine.
Then it responds, "I think you mean: You are the best."
And I feel much better.
—Jack Barry

Nicotine is not my friend. I have absolutely no control over my use of nicotine. I'm an addict. My life became totally unmanageable with my use of nicotine. I was dying, nicotine was killing me. I had no life, except for the death spiral of using. I felt shame and disgust smoking at those feelings and stuffing the feelings back down my throat with each inhale. Then the feeling became even more awful. UGH! I could not stop using. I was spiraling downward in body, mind, and spirit. This is not what I want in my life today!

I had to grieve the loss of my long relationship with nicotine, which was very confusing at the time. I wanted to be free, and yet there was a kind of emptiness which I couldn't quite put my finger on. My sponsor suggested I write a farewell letter to nicotine, and that really helped with facing the addiction and releasing the feelings.

I began to feel better physically, emotionally, and spiritually. This reinforced that feeling good and being happy is what I want in my life today.

---

*Today, help me break the cycle of addiction,
so that I can feel better in my body, mind, and spirit.*

JANUARY 11

No one wants advice—only corroboration.
—John Steinbeck

One of the strengths of this recovery program is the idea that no one really appreciates being told what to do. Our purpose is to offer support, not unsolicited advice or criticism. This is the understanding that I seek at meetings, where I am free to take what I need and leave the rest.

With the guidance I accept from my sponsor and Higher Power, I make choices and even risk potential mistakes. Now I know mistakes are not bad, they are just opportunities to learn and grow. I take responsibility for my own life. I watch, I listen, and notice healthy examples. Members identify with one another rather than compare or judge each other.

We each walk our own path, resisting the temptation to tell other members how they *should* step. We have created a fellowship of mutual support, believing in the slogan, **Together We Change**.

Today, my recovery is a personal process,
which is best shared with others.

JANUARY 12

Each moment can be a fresh start with a fresh breath.
—Nicotine Anonymous Member

Prior to joining NicA, I heard what smoking cessation programs suggested to do to get through a craving. They listed several variations on the 5 Ds: Delay, Distract, Deep breathe, Drink water, Discuss feelings, Develop support, Do something. Those Ds can all be helpful, but such programs offered only temporary support. I needed more, and a solution that continued on for as long as I needed to get free and keep from relapsing.

NicA provides me ongoing support at meetings where I can discuss my feelings without criticism or unsolicited advice. When I began attending, the time during the meeting at least delayed and distracted me for an hour. I could drink water. And, the one D that I always have had with me is a deep breath.

In the past, during a stressful moment my body may have automatically taken a deep breath. However, in NicA, I've come to believe that my deep breaths are my way to make conscious contact with my Higher Power, which brings me into a deep peace. These long, slow deep breaths are now a spiritual experience. The air is the ultimate and necessary connection to life. Each fresh breath gives me a fresh start to live one moment at a time with gratitude for my recovery.

Today, I consciously inhale that which keeps me spiritually inspired.

JANUARY 13

It is the acceptance of our very true and very human limitations.
—Nicotine Anonymous: The Book

When I joined NicA, I had only one desire: to stop smoking. That already seemed too much to ask for. "The Serenity Prayer for Nicotine Users" pamphlet explained I needed to ask for the courage to accept the craving for nicotine. Accept the craving? Initially, I didn't get what that meant. I wanted to get rid of the craving, not accept it. When I tried to accept it, I failed and lit up. I was filled with regret; I believed the craving was more than I could bear.

Members encouraged me to **Keep Showing Up**. I got a sponsor who said I may need to find some serenity first before I could receive the courage I needed. He then suggested I could practice accepting whatever things I could not change during my daily activities. As I did this, I found it calmed me down. I was better at sorting out details and prioritizing my activities. That practice helped me come to believe in the value and purpose of acceptance. My life became more manageable.

I became willing to practice other principles of the program, such as the slogans. They helped me to finally become willing to accept the craving. Days became weeks and I became humbly grateful for my new freedom.

Today, I use our slogan ***Prepare, Practice, Pray, Progress,*** *and find acceptance of myself and others.*

The moment we want to believe something,
we suddenly see all the arguments for it,
and become blind to all the arguments against it.
—George Bernard Shaw

The power of the desire to believe I can use nicotine, convinces me to accept the choices I am making. I do not like to live in doubt. When I was a smoker, I did not want to have doubts about what I was doing. I turned a blind eye to any consequences that raised doubts.

In my youth, tobacco companies' advertising worked to convince me just how good their products were for me. Smoking nicotine provided physical and psychological convincers that blinded me from the truth. To have doubts meant I must be wrong in my beliefs. I couldn't stand for that. So, I was an absolute believer! I became the tyrant of my own tyranny.

Now, in recovery, I can use the power of the desire to live free of nicotine and to believe in the choices I'm making. There is no doubt in this truth. I have admitted I am powerless over nicotine and cleared the air to see my way toward a spiritual awakening. Denial does not blind me any longer; the truth has set me free.

*Today, I am energized by my new beliefs
which make my life more manageable.*

JANUARY 15

If I can accept the craving,
I may learn what it can teach me
—Nicotine Anonymous Member

I've tried to fight the craving. It was exhausting, and ultimately a losing battle. The fight just increased the tension and stress that typically drove me to seek another dose of my drug, nicotine. I was powerless over this addictive substance, and my life was a mess.

I read about accepting the craving in our pamphlet, "The Serenity Prayer for Nicotine Users." That was the first time I had heard of that approach. I'm glad it explained, "Accepting the craving does not mean we want the craving or like it." However, as long as cravings were going to occur, maybe I could improve my attitude about them and learn something from them.

I accepted that I used nicotine, in part, to hide behind a smokescreen. To understand what is hiding behind a craving, I allow myself to be guided by our slogan, **Look for the Lesson**, and to use the tip, **H.A.L.T.** (Hungry, Angry, Lonely, Tired).

The craving could be a signal alerting me to something I actually need or a lesson to learn. Cravings could be very useful for my dulled brain, if I pay attention and respond with more awareness of what my body is telling me as it is healing. But I cannot pay attention by using nicotine. By turning a craving over to my Higher Power, I could find what lies beneath. An old addict can learn new tricks.

Today, I accept the cravings and find the serenity
I have been looking for all along.

JANUARY 16

Neither self-recrimination, willpower,
nor analysis of our situation helped.
—Nicotine Anonymous: The Book

I had often heard the popular wisdom for someone who wanted to quit smoking. Basically, it was, "You have to really want to quit smoking." That usually was followed by, "You have to quit for yourself, not for anybody else." I struggled to care enough to stop and stay stopped for my own sake. Since I was in an insane relationship with nicotine, both loving and hating it, such wisdom did me no good. My shame alone made it difficult to consider myself worthy of self-care. How pitiful was my insufficient willpower I thought necessary to quit this habit.

On my own, I just couldn't tap into enough inner care. When I discovered a NicA meeting, I half wanted help, and half thought I may need more humiliation to motivate me out of my usual behaviors and thought patterns. The usual tools of self-recrimination, my own feeble willpower, and analytical mind were useless. No wonder my life was unmanageable.

The group accepted me with my tenuous little desire. They gave me their encouraging care each week. I realized I needed a care greater than myself. I finally admitted my powerlessness and gave in to giving up nicotine, mostly because I cared about the people in my group. Eventually, I felt worthy enough to truly care about my own wellbeing.

---

*Today, in recovery, I take good care of myself for my own sake
and for those who care about me.*

JANUARY 17

Divine Grace please help me, I cannot do this alone.
—Nicotine Anonymous Member

Coming to terms with my nicotine addiction was a process for me. At first, I was only able to say, "I should stop, but not yet." This was a dash of honesty, but it didn't move me to humility. In time I said, "Oh, I wish I could stop, but it's too hard to do." I was feeling the desire to stop, but wishing is not yet willing to stop. Eventually I felt the confused desperation of, "Oh my God, I give up! I'm willing to do anything!"

In that dark isolated moment, I decided to search on the web. I found the Nicotine Anonymous website. I read the Twelve Steps and I was somewhat concerned about the references to God. Although I believed in sacredness, I wondered if Nicotine Anonymous was a cult. There wasn't a meeting near me, but I saw that there were internet meetings, so I attended one.

At first, I just listened. Someone shared that his understanding of G.O.D. meant Grace Of Divinity. Then others shared their spiritual understanding of a Power greater than themselves, and how this understanding was helping them with their recovery. Each held to their own individual beliefs, but also were united as a community with a common purpose. That worked for me.

Today, I am willing to ask for and accept Divine Grace as a powerful source of help.

JANUARY 18

Life only demands from you the strength that you possess.
Only one feat is possible; not to run away.

—Dag Hammarskjold

For me, nicotine was not only a way of deadening emotions and internal reactions, but also a way to try to stop outside demands from coming in. Nicotine gave me an illusion of control that I could manage the pace of the constant interplay of internal and external forces that demanded my attention. In truth, my life was out of control and my use of nicotine completely unmanageable.

As smoking-related health threats increased, I realized that this deadening also blocked my increasing desire to stop smoking from seeing a way out of my nicotine fog. Then, I found a NicA meeting where we are asked to listen to others' experiences, and not interrupt, gossip, or offer unsolicited advice. This became the safe space I so desperately wanted. Prior to coming to meetings, I had not known how to create it without the use of nicotine.

I still struggle with responding to the constant bombardment of stimuli from both the outside world and my inner world. However, my meeting is a refuge that also shows me how to create a safe place in my life without using nicotine or doing other compulsive behaviors.

Today, I will deal with life's demands by accepting that all I need to do is the next right thing.

JANUARY 19

However early you get up, you cannot hasten the dawn.
—Spanish Proverb

I bought all the literature and read it all through. I showed up early for meetings. After several weeks I was still smoking. I was impatient and doubtful the program would work for me. But what else could I do? So, I kept listening and got a sponsor.

I heard that recovery is a process whose pace may not seem fast enough to please me. I can work this program diligently, but it doesn't mean I can make things happen as fast as I want. My sponsor told me that her process unfolded just the way it was necessary for her, not the way she wanted, but the way she needed. She felt her recovery process was guided by a Power greater than herself.

I was looking for a quick fix, just as smoking had been. I have thought of myself as clever, and typically look for short cuts or an easier way.

Recovery is not an area where such cleverness is an asset. For me, patience is an aspect of faith. Patience allows me time to process things on a deeper level, in ways to become completely willing to let go. If I want to learn all I can from this program, I find there is more that I need to let go of than just my cigarettes.

Today, I ask for the wisdom to know how patience will make my life more manageable.

JANUARY 20

Sometimes I feel so vulnerable that anyone's wrong word at me could cause me to relapse back to nicotine.

—Nicotine Anonymous Member

I admitted to my addiction when I went without my constant doses of nicotine. Those first days seemed like months. Although they were some of the most painful, I do not want to forget them, lest I relapse. Sometimes withdrawal felt like teetering on a tightrope, or having molten lava bubbling at the brim, or walking on my own egg shells. The process of getting free of the toxins felt like someone had turned up my emotions' sensitivity to the maximum. I felt skinless and vulnerable. I did not know if I wanted to scream, rant, or cry. There was nowhere to hide, nowhere to run, except to my NicA meeting.

The acceptance and support I found at meetings allowed me a safe place to talk about these difficult feelings. At first, I was either afraid or embarrassed to have others know my true feelings. I took comfort from *Nicotine Anonymous: The Book* saying I was "not awful," and that I would be "humbled to realize that [I was] normal—and just very human."

Although words can trigger me, I do not have to react by dosing up. I have help, so I have hope. Through my fellow members, I have the words of this program, and I am coming to believe they are all part of a Power greater than myself.

Today, I will soothe my raw edges with the gentle care of a Power greater than myself.

JANUARY 21

Even if you're on the right track,
you'll get run over if you just sit there.
—Will Rogers

When I came to Nicotine Anonymous meetings, I was still using nicotine. However, I felt like I was in a comfortable, safe place. To contribute service, I helped with the readings in NicA meetings. I waited my turn to share. I admitted my continuing use of nicotine. I humbly apologized.

On days between meetings, I did not change anything. I didn't read the literature. I didn't call another member. I didn't seek out a sponsor. I took comfort in just attending the meeting. I was told I could take the program at my own pace. I continued to use nicotine at my own pace, quite a lot, and with a nervous, insatiable discontent. NicA had wrecked my smoking.

In time, I came face to face with the fatal attraction and admitted my powerlessness. In truth, I sought comfort in appearing to do something, when really I was doing as little as possible, while slowly killing myself. That's basically what smoking is: appearing busy when doing nothing and dying slowly. Nicotine Anonymous provided me the right track. I needed to blow the whistle and get rolling.

Today, I seek comfort in positive action;
I reach out, and create hope.

JANUARY 22

Every dawn signs a new contract with existence.
—Henri Frederic Amiel

No matter what my past behavior was, each day begins with a fresh opportunity to exercise my spiritual muscles. Yes, sometimes mountainous cravings will appear, and obsession may steal my strength. I use this program to prepare for such situations, which gives me the willingness and courage to pedal on up the hills. With recovery, I learn I have choices to change my course and my attitude.

I started using as a child, before I learned how to make choices about my behavior. While actively using nicotine as I grew up, the fact that I had a choice to change did not seem real. Addiction warped my reality and robbed my options. I just reacted to the moment. Emotionally stunted by nicotine, I never developed the healthy skills required to respond to life in mature ways. I just reached for a cigarette to cope. No wonder my life was unmanageable.

Now, with this program and a Higher Power, I begin to make new and healthier choices that each new day offers me. With each dawn, I also make a new commitment to work this program and build my spiritual strength.

Coasting only works if I'm heading down hill. If I want to get somewhere, I need to be pedaling. My Higher Power's wind is upon my back helping me face the hills that will come.

Today, I build strong spiritual muscles,
and respond to life in healthy, mature ways.

JANUARY 23

The need for change bulldozed a road down my mind.
—Maya Angelou

After years of nicotine use, my soul screamed for relief and comfort from the insidiousness of nicotine addiction. But, reaching out for help outside myself has always been an issue. Aren't I a capable human being? Haven't I solved other important problems with little input from anyone else? Then why is Nicotine Anonymous always suggesting to use telephone lists or get a sponsor?

Those in the fellowship have learned something that I pray to be open enough to experience: asking for help. Relying even slightly on another human being makes me accountable to someone else. It also keeps me accountable to my word.

Reaching out to someone else teaches me the value of humility. So, I ask myself, am I still teachable? After all, if I could do this myself, why am I still struggling? If I can take that very tiny first step and humbly ask for help, doing so might just save my life.

Today, I reach out for help
and I find relief and comfort.

JANUARY 24

Life had begun to feel as if I were standing up in a canoe.
—Nicotine Anonymous Member

Admitting my life was unmanageable was rather easy. I was continually trying to balance reality and fantasy, sanity and insanity. No matter which direction I turned, I was struggling against the current without a paddle. I didn't know how much longer I could stand it, much less stand up, before tipping over. I was on the verge of drowning in the chaos of trying to numb myself or hide behind a cloud of smoke.

My NicA group gave me a place to set my anchor and steady myself. That helped me let go of nicotine, but the currents still swirled around me. I had a series of deaths among family and friends, which were deeply painful and brought up emotional wounds from my earlier life. I had a slip and smoked while trying to avoid feeling these emotions, and quickly realized that nicotine didn't work for me anymore. I shared this at my next meeting and felt some relief in my fellow addicts' care.

Care is what I need to soothe and heal pains, old and new. A sponsor, a therapist, and an additional support group: all are under consideration. It's time to make some new decisions.

Today, I pray for the knowledge and power of love from Good Orderly Direction.

JANUARY 25

I was just a kid, half-baked, half-brained,
and acting in half-assed ways most of the time.
—Nicotine Anonymous Member

I was susceptible to becoming a nicotine addict as a teenager because I wanted to control my emotions or avoid feeling them. I have learned that the emotional part of a teen's brain is fully developed, but the intellect and reasoning center does not fully develop until the mid-twenties. My half-brained response to justify putting toxic substances in my body was made of a long list of excuses and lies.

By the time I had a fully developed brain, I was deep into the jungle of justifications for my addiction. To reconcile the insanity, I imagined and believed in false realities. The chemical addiction and compulsive behavior were like quicksand. The more I smoked, the deeper I sank. It took a really low bottom before I reached out for help.

Nicotine Anonymous meetings eased me back to reality, because I could listen and talk without the need to defend myself with excuses and justifications. I heard hope and truth sitting courageously beside me. My group threw me a lifeline, and fortunately I finally had the good sense to grab it.

Today, I leave the jungle quicksand behind
and become an emotionally mature adult.

JANUARY 26

There are no accidents.
Consider, as I learned to do,
the incredible interconnectedness of life.
—Wayne Dyer

My actions create a series of consequences, each influencing the next in some way. Even when I am in denial, these events influence my self- esteem.

When I was active in my addiction, I thought that what I did to myself didn't matter. I was an adult and I could do whatever I wanted, right? If I didn't die immediately after using nicotine, could it really be that bad?

My actions created unmanageable situations, which lessened my opinion of myself, creating a perpetual cycle of insanity. By working the Twelve Steps, I have come to understand that my ill-at-ease responses to the realities of life were immature.

In recovery, I am discovering the connectedness between my own power and the greater power of the God of my understanding. I am learning that my thoughts and actions affect me and others in my life.

Physicists have learned that everything exists only in relationship to everything else; nothing can exist separately. Working the Twelve Steps helps me to align myself more with our interconnectedness.

Today, I see how my thoughts and actions matter,
as I see the incredible interconnectedness of life.

JANUARY 27

From childhood, we were taught to rely on ourselves.
We learned that no one was going to do it for us.
—Nicotine Anonymous: The Book

We think we don't need help, but we always do. When I first joined Nicotine Anonymous, it was a challenge for me to even begin to seek or ask for help. I resisted because I was afraid to expose any lack of ability that would leave me vulnerable to criticism or ridicule. I also believed that short of being locked in a rubber room, no one could help me stop smoking. It didn't make sense that someone else could do something for me that I could not do for myself. Clearly, for years I could not stop myself.

By attending meetings and reading our literature, I began to see that asking for help was an act of strength, not weakness. I surrendered and became willing to try anything, which included allowing others and a Higher Principle, as something good and wonderful, to help and guide me.

I came to understand that NicA is not about any so-called self-help method. Instead, it is about mutual support: we help each other. At the end of life there are no awards presented for persevering alone or choosing the hard road.

Today, I choose the easier path of mutual support where rewards are here and now.

JANUARY 28

I have always felt that doubt was the beginning of wisdom.
—Clarence Darrow

As a newcomer, I entered my first Nicotine Anonymous meeting with arms folded and all sorts of attitudes. I came with doubts. I expected to have things to complain about and nitpick over. I have come to realize those attitudes were an attempt to protect myself from my expectation of failing to stop smoking.

Like many nicotine addicts, I have boundary issues. I am uncertain where and how I fit in this world. In the beginning, nicotine use was a way for me to become part of one group while it separated me from another. As a child, I didn't have permission to say no and have that honored. As an adult, I had lived with the difficulty of saying no when I needed to.

I used my smoke to create a boundary around me. It may have been my rebellious way of saying no. The honesty of this recovery program helps me see how I resist and to understand the why of my resistance.

The wisdom I ask for in the Serenity Prayer helps me to know when I should say no and when I should say yes. There's a time to let my guard down, as well as to put it up. Recovery brings clarity to move forward with healthy boundaries.

Today, my spiritual surrender allows me
to avoid where I don't need to go
and shows me where I want to be.

JANUARY 29

It was a gut-wrenching coming to terms with the fact
that we were hooked on a drug.

—Nicotine Anonymous: The Book

I felt that wrench keep tightening in my gut for years. On my own, I just couldn't come to terms with breaking up this dysfunctional relationship. Nicotine's control, for me, was absolute and without mercy.

I wanted to end the madness, but I could not get a handle on the wrench to loosen the nicotine nut. Yet, I soothed myself with nutty ideas that sucking in all those toxins would not harm me, as if I was immune to its diseases.

At the NicA meeting, I heard each week, "…if we want to be free of nicotine, we need to become willing to go to any length. This program offers us a way to reach our goal." It became clear that I had to come at this from deep in my gut. I would need to be all in and totally committed. No more nutty ideas or magical thinking allowed. I had to grow up, take responsibility, and be accountable.

On a gut level, I humbly surrendered, admitted my powerlessness, and became completely open to receive caring support. I needed a power greater than nicotine. I was willing to endure the discomfort of withdrawal and trust the program's promised benefits. My fellow members' experience, strength, and hope supported me. Now, I return that caring support to newcomers. I breathe, do good work, and help others.

---

*Today, I fulfill my needs by doing the things I need to do
for the maintenance of my recovery.*

JANUARY 30

The wolf will hire himself out very cheaply as a shepherd.
—Russian Proverb

Before recovery, I believed the lie that nicotine is a solution to all sorts of things. Advertisements convinced me that using nicotine would make me feel cool and calm, satisfied with pleasure, admired, and accepted. I was influenced by these lies, and I ignored the dangers. I got caught up in the illusion that I was getting something.

In the real world, nicotine doesn't give me anything worth the price, and I have paid plenty. It has no nutritional value or any real benefits, nor can it make me into somebody. Nicotine is just a useless addictive substance. Any satisfaction is more a relief that comes from temporarily feeding a craving that keeps instigating the next craving.

In the end it's all smoke. There's nothing to get except a filthy ashtray, but there is so much to lose.

The principles of this recovery program are my new shepherds. This is a gentle program that offers, asks, suggests, and supports me to discover a greater shepherd of my own understanding. Members are respected as individuals, but are united in our primary purpose to help each other live free from nicotine.

Today, I am guided to real satisfaction.
I find inner pleasure and freedom.

Surrender is a gift that you can give yourself. It's an act of faith.
It's saying that even though I can't see where this river is flowing,
I trust it will take me in the right direction.

—Debbie Ford

Getting to the point of total and utter surrender by thoroughly working Step One is what helped me set my quit date and practice the 5 D's more often. It began with the willingness to be willing. A shred of my Higher Power's grace filtered through my insanity during meetings. And I worked Step Two. I read "The Serenity Prayer for Nicotine Users" pamphlet over and over.

As I was leaping empty-handed into what seemed like the scary place of not knowing how to cope without nicotine, I was totally supported by my friends in NicA and my Higher Power. I did not curl up and die, I did not run screaming naked down the street with my hair on fire. Nothing happened. Cravings came, I asked my HP for help, and I asked members of my group for help through the cravings. The cravings came and went. Life went on. I still had to deal with myself and my reactions to life.

My NicA group and my HP's unconditional love supported me while I worked on my shortcomings. My sponsor helped me clarify my character assets, and to see my part in the wreckage of my past. As I continued to surrender, I forgave, accepted and even began loving myself.

The Steps provide a path and the Traditions the guidelines for dealing with life on life's terms. Today, I keep it simple, breathe, surrender, and do the next right thing.

Today, I let go and experience the miracle of freedom from nicotine.

We saw our own insanity—
repeating the same actions over and over,
expecting the results to be different.
—Nicotine Anonymous: The Book

I don't want to feel crazy or knowingly ingest poison. If I keep hitting my head against the wall and it hurts, I should stop hitting my head against the wall, right? Aside from the spiritual malady and the phenomenon of craving, it was always the peculiar mental twist that precedes the first cigarette, over which I was powerless.

I knew the difference between right and wrong; it was the primary reason for my guilt and shame. Doing the same thing over and over, and each time expecting a different result is the insanity of this addiction. Like when I promised myself to have just one, and well, you all know what happens then. Like all the times it happened again and again and again, all the months and years I continued to do the same thing, each time expecting a different result.

What could restore me to sanity? Step Two says, "...a Power greater than ourselves..." Belief is the key—If I believe a chair will hold me up, then I sit in that chair. If I believe that the God of my understanding will help me get free from my addiction, then I seek my Higher Power's strength and have faith. Believing that my HP loves me and is bigger than my addiction, is a powerful step toward recovery.

I need something powerful enough for my mind to discern that nicotine is a lethal poison, so I never choose to take that first puff.

Today, I know that without help, getting free of nicotine
is too powerful of a task for me alone,
so, I turn to a Power greater than myself.

Just how insane does it have to get?
—Nicotine Anonymous Member

It once seemed normal to smoke two packs of cigarettes a day. I would hear about all the dangers of lung disease and death, but think that I was somehow special and immune to such consequences. Sometimes I would smoke in the shower and think that I was clever. If I ran out of cigarettes, going out to the store—no matter the time, distance, or weather—was just something I had to do.

When I caught a cold or the flu, I only smoked what I thought was a reasonable number of cigarettes. Doing so may have delayed getting better, but again, I considered it acceptable. When a doctor informed me I was developing chronic lung disease, I switched to so-called light cigarettes. But the coughing and chest pains did not improve.

A friend told me about Nicotine Anonymous and urged me to check it out. It sounded a bit crazy, a support group to stop smoking? How could other people help me with that?

I heard members who had stopped smoking share past experiences that were similar to mine. Listening to others honestly

admit to their own crazy behaviors, I began to honestly admit mine. I began to realize all the ways my life had become unmanageable due to the insanity of nicotine addiction. Instead of shame, I felt relief.

Today, I wake up with hope,
and I see sanity looking at me in the mirror.

FEBRUARY 3

To feel that one has a place in life
solves half the problem of contentment.
—George E. Woodberry

As long as I ingested nicotine into my body, I rejected the chance for real contentment. How was I going to feel contentment when I was compulsively sucking in toxins, self-loathing, and worry? When I felt unsafe, my mind sought protection from my disturbing reality. Denial kept me from seeing that the way I was seeking protection was actually harmful to me!

In addition to the emotional distress, there was also the time and money spent on my addiction. The many potential pleasures and achievements that I missed made for resentments. There is no real contentment in a life full of resentments.

When I found my way to a meeting, I found a home where experience, strength, and hope are shared. Once I began my recovery and got clean, I began to feel gratitude. Gratitude is a gateway to peace. After spending years abusing myself in the endless cycle of craving due to my use of nicotine, I am now seeking saner ways to feel contentment. Meetings have become a place where I can feel I belong. I am safe to relax and celebrate my achievement—I am content.

Today, my Nicotine Anonymous meeting
is a place for contentment.

FEBRUARY 4

It is a very rare mind that believes what it does,
and does what it actually believes. But only in such a mind are
thought, feeling, and action really one.
—A. R. Orage

Living as a nicotine addict is like having an axe that's continually splitting my sanity apart from my actions. There is just no sanity to the action of ingesting poisonous and carcinogenic chemical compounds into my body. Whether I admit it or not, this addiction enslaves me into continual conflict. Denial may blind me of the war, but the battle rages and the losses mount.

Recovery from this disease can return me to a more harmonious state of being. Yes, it can be challenging to believe in what I do and to do what I believe. However, the task is eased as I recover from this disease.

When I stop creating a continuous conflict by repeatedly consuming nicotine, I have an opportunity for peace. With peace I can make amends and rebuild my belief and trust in myself.

I no longer run away from my feelings, so I get clearer about what I believe. The peace of mind that comes from this spiritual surrender allows my thoughts, feelings, and actions to come together into one presence.

Today, I am more in sync with my belief.
I draw on the strength of my inner integrity to guide my actions.

We are so blind
To all the realm of real, so numb to feeling
Anything but the ache inside the breast,
It takes a miracle to make the healing
Miracle of beauty manifest.
—Alfred Barret

I spent years refusing to take an honest look at my addiction. The longer the years, the more I longed to feel better. But how could I when nicotine only gave me spikes of relief, then deadness—nothing good would last.

The daily consequences of using were subtle at first. Then bronchitis kept recurring and I became less and less active. As smoke-free laws were passed, it was no longer cool to smoke, and I became more isolated. Yet even when these signs appeared, I was so deep into my addiction, I believed I could not escape.

Then one day I stopped at a diner and noticed a former acquaintance sitting in a booth. We got to chatting. I was coughing and he shared how he had found recovery by going to Nicotine Anonymous meetings. I remember saying, "It would take a miracle for me to stop smoking." His story was inspiring, so I began by checking out NicA meetings on the internet. It wasn't long before I wanted to be restored to sanity more than I wanted to smoke.

This program suggests that I become open to a miracle, an event not of my own making. I had always considered myself self-reliant, but I've finally admitted self-reliance wasn't working to get free of nicotine. I needed a Power greater than myself, yes, a miracle, to restore me to sanity.

Today, I work my program and I am getting my miracle.

FEBRUARY 6

There are wounds that cannot be medicated.
—Nicotine Anonymous Member

Through the ages, seemingly impossible struggles and violations have challenged so many people. Often those who endured and even triumphed over these experiences did so because of a personal spirituality they had come to believe in. Personal spirituality has a power to transcend brute force and elevate us above deep longing.

As a nicotine addict, I was confronted with the brute nicotine, and longed for years to be free of its choke hold. I wrestled with my problem intellectually and emotionally, day after day.

I accept that I have wounds that cannot be medicated away with nicotine. In recovery, I find relief using my own personal spiritual remedy and daily practice. At meetings, I witness others receiving this healing as we come to believe that a Power greater than ourselves can restore us to sanity. It is this kind of spiritual H.E.L.P. which Heals Every Longing Person.

Today, my remedy comes from taking the Steps
toward my own personal spirituality.

FEBRUARY 7

Go outside, to the fields, enjoy nature and the sunshine,
go out and try to recapture happiness in yourself and in God.
Think of all the beauty that's still left
in and around you and be happy
—Anne Frank

I could recall, as a young child, enjoying nature and playing sports, a happiness I felt before I started smoking. Growing older, my days were busy, but a lot of time was consumed by the behaviors of my addiction. I didn't spend much time stopping to smell the roses, in part, because smoking deadened my sense of smell.

So absorbed in feeding my addiction, when smoking indoors, I was in a dark, hopeless place no matter how much light there may have been. When outdoors, I left my toxic butts wherever I took my last drag, totally oblivious that I used nature as my ashtray.

The first time I read Step Two in *Nicotine Anonymous: The Book*, I was almost moved to tears when I read about "a willingness to allow something good to happen to ourselves." I've come to realize that allowing for even a glimmer of hope is an activity, not a passive waiting.

Now I seek and embrace inspiration in the beauty of nature. I take slow walks in the woods to notice the variety of life forms. I lie on beach sands to listen to the ocean as its waves soothe me with their ancient song. I climb hills to gape in awe at the vista.

When I focus on what is beautiful in my life and on my spiritual path, I raise my sights to a higher attitude.

Today, I take time to go where the beauty is
and let it lift my spirits to where joy abounds!

FEBRUARY 8

What we fear of doing most is usually what we most need to do.
—Ralph Waldo Emerson

Fear is generally a defensive reaction against change from what's familiar. Resistance, by any other name, smells just as problematic. During my first months at meetings, I joined with members each week reciting the Serenity Prayer. After some time, I realized how valuable the prayer was—to restore me to sanity—in order to better manage my daily life.

Fear and resistance were instinctive reflexes to a threat to my comfort. Smoking for so many years created familiarity and comfort. Changing that familiar comfort felt threatening, even though I knew smoking is deadly. Thinking about the actual toxic threat in smoke just made me even more uncomfortable. Satisfying the urgent need for immediate, familiar comfort ruled each moment. In NicA meetings I felt a new sense of comfort which calmed my fears.

As members shared the benefits of changing their resistance to quitting, I asked to be granted the same courage—to change the things I most needed to change. With the inspiration of my fellow members, I let go of my resistance. I now feel safe to make the transition to a new familiarity with recovery.

Today, I act with new courage to do what I most need to do.

FEBRUARY 9

Out of the despair and without understanding why,
there came an awareness of an alternative.
We accepted the possibility of hope.
—Nicotine Anonymous: The Book

I came to my first meeting with despair in my heart. If I couldn't do it myself, I didn't believe anything or anyone could get me to stop using nicotine. I was convinced I couldn't break away from this drug that had me in its jaws.

With no better options, I made a commitment to keep going to meetings each week. Looking back, my attendance revealed an awareness of an alternative. I could have stayed home and kept using nicotine. Now, I had an alternative for an hour a week.

Another alternative was to actually listen to other members who were either still struggling or who were enjoying their freedom. I could have dismissed them with a good-for-them attitude, but I didn't. Then I accepted a service role. That too was an alternative to just coming to the meeting and then leaving.

Over time, my progress with this process helped me believe I had an alternative to despair: hope. Through making new choices, I came to believe in the possibilities of freedom from nicotine.

Today, I accept the possibility of hope.

FEBRUARY 10

Even the ignorant man knows when
an ill-fitting shoe is pinching his foot.
—Anonymous

Breathing air is basic to grounding oneself and supporting life. As a smoker, I had gotten used to taking a deep drag on a cigarette. Trying to breathe without nicotine for any length of time seemed so strange and even impossible. The whole idea was discomforting.

Now, that seems insane, doesn't it? I think anybody who has not been addicted to nicotine can clearly see just how insane this belief is. I didn't know how to breathe without nicotine. I believed that to live without nicotine, I would have to learn how to breathe again.

The level of denial necessary to maintain my addiction to nicotine was the thing that stopped me from doing anything really constructive about it. After attending a number of meetings, I could see how much this basic life affirming human activity—breathing—had gotten so complicated during my nicotine use. I found saying the Serenity Prayer was like getting a dose from an oxygen mask when stressed out or unable to focus due to anxiety.

When I was a smoker, I met discomfort with just another drag. Recovery has shown me how a feeling of discomfort can tell me when something is off kilter. I can acknowledge my discomfort without having to breathe in nicotine to numb myself out from what is really bothering me. In doing so, I can practice behaviors that are truly helpful for me, because the feeling will pass whether I smoke or not.

Today, I breathe in all the fresh air I possibly can.

FEBRUARY 11

When I took a puff, I was trying to draw in
some serenity, courage, or wisdom out of a lit stick.
—Nicotine Anonymous Member

Recovery is about learning to make new choices and take new steps to change the direction of my life. Even though I accept I am powerless over nicotine, I am not helpless. Even though I accept I have cravings set off by physical and psychological triggers, I don't have to respond by using nicotine. As I learn about new choices, I can practice new ways of meeting my needs and being content.

I have a disease of the body and mind. The Twelve Steps offer me a spiritual solution which helps me to be free from this imprisoning drug. The Steps suggest a way to develop my own spiritual nature, to sensing a powerful force that is more than just me. This conscious spiritual contact provides me with the serenity, courage, and wisdom which helps me do what I could not do on my own.

Now, in recovery, I find a better way. I make progress when I **Prepare, Practice, Pray, Progress**, instead of puffing my life away.

Today, I practice making new choices
and being happy, joyous, and free.

FEBRUARY 12

The best time to plant a tree was 20 years ago.
The second-best time is now.
—Chinese proverb

I regretted using nicotine for the last 20 years of my addiction. I knew nicotine was dangerous. It bothered me that my money went to the nicotine industry's profits. It was an insane absurdity to be paying someone else to kill me. I did this to myself.

When I heard about a local Nicotine Anonymous meeting, I joined. I struggled for months during my quest to gain freedom from this beast. With the group's support, I finally surrendered and began to be restored to sanity.

Yet, once I experienced the daily reprieve as an actual reality, I had remorse that I hadn't done it sooner. This remorse poisoned the joy I wanted to feel about gaining my freedom. With more meetings, and saying the Serenity Prayer, I forgave myself. The remorse was lifted, and I began to live more in the present. I accepted that I cannot change the past.

My past insanity led me to NicA and the gift of recovery from this insidious addiction. Becoming a committed member has improved my life beyond what I had ever imagined. Our slogan, **Look for the Lesson**, guides me to take from my experiences what is valuable, and leave the rest.

Today, I live in the present, and am the best I can be right now.

FEBRUARY 13

Getting real is the only deal!
—Nicotine Anonymous Member

From the time I saw my first cigarette commercial, I was under the influence of an illusion. The cowboy was a rugged individualist, the James Bond character was cool, and menthol was that fresh country taste. In reality, these qualities had no real relationship to tobacco and the consequences of using it.

Living with painful cancer or coronary disease, or gasping for air from having emphysema are the reality for many nicotine users. I lived for years with the illusion that it was somehow different for me. I wanted to believe the illusion because if I didn't, I was left with only the insanity of constant cravings and lame rationalizations.

My recovery is based on honesty and owning up to the consequences of my actions. I look at reality and face the denial. I practice the Twelve Steps as a process to ease me forward through my recovery, to come out of the illusion and step into reality. These Steps have saved so many lives. They work if I work them. That I am certain is real!

Today, I let go of my wheelin' and dealin' with the truth,
and accept that getting real is the only deal.

FEBRUARY 14

Success is the sum of small efforts,
repeated day in and day out.
—Robert Collier

Before joining Nicotine Anonymous, my belief about getting free of nicotine was, "It's impossible." But if it ever was possible, it would be like flipping a switch. I would go from using nicotine to not using, and that would be that. My problem was, I couldn't do "that."

Listening at meetings, reading NicA literature, I learned "that" was not how it works. Our pamphlet "How Nicotine Anonymous Works" tells us that Honesty, Openness, and Willingness are essential principles that create a pathway to gain that freedom from nicotine.

On that pathway, there are Steps to take, truths to admit, attitudes to let go, and behaviors to change. I came to understand that recovery is not an on/off event. It's a process of being open and willing to make even small efforts to move forward. I wasn't ready to do the mile, but I could do an inch or a foot. Each effort I made added up to a new strength and courage to reach that place I longed for: to be happy, joyous, and free, living without nicotine.

---

*Today, I make even small efforts
to move forward along my spiritual pathway.*

FEBRUARY 15

When the solution is simple, God is answering.
—Albert Einstein

If I focus on the problem, it gnaws at me like a dog with a bare bone and nothing to gain. Without a recovery program, I only knew my problem, the insanity. With the Second Step, I introduced myself to the solution of being restored to sanity, to having the full life I wanted. When I focus on the solution, I am drawn toward it and away from the problem.

In the beginning of my recovery, Step Two was a process of coming to believe in hope. As I improved my conscious contact through the Steps and the fellowship, I came to believe that the program itself is a Power greater than me. I now see this is how so many are becoming free and living free from nicotine.

Recovery is a process to ease what gnaws at me and has more in store for me than just being free of nicotine. I now have a valuable solution I can share with my fellow addicts who yearn to be free. My desire to get nicotine free has turned into a strong passion to stay nicotine free. I practice new attitudes and behaviors so I can be fully present for what matters in my life.

Today, I have hope because
I stay focused on the solution.

FEBRUARY 16

I came to believe in mysterious capacities to change
when I became willing to go to any length.

—Nicotine Anonymous Member

My experience in recovery has been to witness a miraculous power lift the human spirit. As so many have shared, there was a rebirth at a moment of excruciating pain and desperation. This birth remains a wondrous event. Before recovery, I didn't see pain as potential or a dead end as opportunity. Now I do.

Recovery has offered me a new way to view life. I needed to reach a physical, emotional, and spiritual bottom before I could honestly begin climbing upward. It took reaching this bottom to finally surrender and humbly ask for help. Listening to other members I understood that left to my own ways, I would not get free of nicotine.

The gift came when, inspired by my fellow members, my closed mind opened up to my capacity to change. I accepted the program's suggestion that I needed to be willing to go to any length. Once I became that willing, I found that I didn't need to go as far as I had thought to increase my capacity to change.

When I work this program of recovery, I make conscious contact with a powerful life source. I become more connected to my mysterious capacities to change beyond my wildest dreams.

Today, I have the courage and willingness to open my mind and reach toward the best version of myself.

I used cigarettes to take the edge off all my emotions, including nervousness, fear, love, stress, and even happiness.

—Nicotine Anonymous: The Book

Even happiness? How sad. It once seemed to make sense to use nicotine to relieve stress. That edginess of urgency caused me to notice my frantic grasps for my pack and lighter. That frenzy was as if I was trying to catch my breath when, in truth, I was losing it. Yet, the common belief among smokers was that nicotine relieved stress and therefore was justified, something needed. It would take NicA meetings and reading the science to enlighten me that lighting up actually created stress.

But relieve happiness? What? I couldn't even manage happiness without nicotine? Facing that fact while reading Rodger's Story was to take "a daring look deep into the mirror." My insanity thought I couldn't be happy if I stopped using nicotine, that nicotine even enhanced happiness. Yet, my nicotine use was a constant source of shame. Fear and confusion were driven by withdrawal symptoms I mostly thought of as reminders that it was time for a smoke.

How would I replace that misguided source of happiness? In Rodger's Story he writes, "I have been given so much physically, emotionally, and spiritually from this program...I continue to go to meetings and be of service." I found my answer.

Today, I experience a spiritual happiness by gratefully showing up and offering service.

FEBRUARY 18

Mystery creates wonder
and wonder is the basis of man's desire to understand.
—Neil Armstrong

The essence of our very existence is a mystery far greater than our own understanding. What creates the pulse of life that makes our hearts beat and our lungs breathe?

As I become conscious, every second I experience awe and humility in this amazing life. The only way to resolve the matters which cause me suffering is by coming to believe a Power greater than myself can and will restore me to sanity. This gives me hope, which grows faith. Faith is a common feature of human nature which inspires gratitude, awe and wonder.

Worlds of intricate life and the ever-expanding cosmos are way beyond what an entire history of humans has been able to explain or even grasp. Yet, as I make conscious contact with life in this one moment, I stand in wonder of it all. I don't lie to myself or shy away from being fully present by using nicotine.

My existence is often a mystery to me and beyond my human understanding. The Power that I have come to believe in inspires great wonder and amazement as it creates the pulse of life here within me and all around me. I offer gratitude for this extraordinary gift, especially my next nicotine-free breath.

Today, I am in awe of the wonder of life,
and I embrace the mystery.

Remember that there was a time
when you could live without that thing or that person—
nothing is irreplaceable, a habit is not a need.
—Paulo Coelho

After I got past the grief about leaving behind my faithful little sidekicks, I began to consider the cost of my years of addiction. Not to get depressed, but to get a clearer idea about what I had given up.

There was the money spent buying nicotine over 27 years. Then I added the time spent going to get it, using it, searching for where I last left my stash, and looking for the paraphernalia. How about the time my mind spent spinning either about how to get somewhere to smoke or to quit smoking?

How many days were wasted with respiratory diseases? The salary lost? How many pieces of furniture or articles of clothing got burn holes? Then there were the close calls I had while driving distracted, fumbling for my pack or dropping a lit ash into my lap. I don't even know if I may have started a brush fire by flicking butts out my car window.

How many things did I not do for lack of breath? What people and places did I avoid? The physical, mental, emotional, and spiritual toll on my life was staggering. When I consider how much this disease has taken from me, I realize the grand hoax: I "haven't given up anything at all."

Today, I am blessed with a whole new life nicotine-free.
I make new choices with my new found freedom.

FEBRUARY 20

When I identify with others, I connect.
When I compare myself with others, I separate.
—Nicotine Anonymous Member

In recovery, I identify with my fellows' goals to stop using nicotine and to benefit from using the Twelve Steps. The program guides me away from getting caught up in comparison-making. We may have our different experiences, but making comparisons usually leads to judgments.

My smoking began at age 12 in part, because of my low self-esteem based on comparing myself to others. My judgments usually became an exercise in unfair injustice toward others or myself.

Comparisons put the focus on differences and they separate me from others. I've come to see that if I compare myself with others, it's either to lower myself into a familiar pity pit, or to lower others just so I feel better for a while. Comparing leads to resentments, not remedies.

When I allow myself to be open and identify my similarities with others, there is an opportunity for insight and growth. When I share how we are similar, I connect and create a bond with others, and I develop compassion and respect for others.

Today, I practice finding our similarities,
and I seek ways to connect with others.

It is best in the theatre to act with confidence,
no matter how little right you have to it.
—Lillian Hellman

Whenever I had thoughts about giving up nicotine, I did not have confidence about quitting. The disease of addiction robbed me of my confidence and self-worth. Each time I used, my confidence and conviction to change my destructive behavior was further damaged.

However, when I began attending Nicotine Anonymous meetings, I heard I could "act as if." Although I felt afraid to change my behavior, I could act as if I were brave. I may not be able to see myself as successful, but maybe I can imagine myself as someone who is.

When my quit date arrived, it helped to act as if I could delay lighting up. Now, when I face a character defect I'm scared to change, I know I can act as if I can work through it. I accept that I am making an attempt, even if only for a few moments, and begin to build confidence. I can take things one step at a time.

This is a gentle program. I only look for progress, not perfection, even if I am just "acting as if" for this moment. Action encourages hope. As I make progress to change the things I can, I restore my self-confidence, one small action at a time.

Today, I "act as if" and take action,
I am confident to move forward in my recovery.

FEBRUARY 22

I don't know how I can trust my Higher Power
when I'm driving. What does God know about driving a car?
—Nicotine Anonymous Member

It was difficult for me to get comfortable with a Higher Power of my own understanding. I grew up with some religion, which was centered in a church. My previous concept of a god belonged only in church, which sometimes was a positive experience for me, sometimes it wasn't. God was separate from my everyday activities such as my job, caring for my children, or driving my car. My daily activities just seemed like my business; God had bigger stuff to do.

Caught up in the insanity of my addiction, it was difficult to believe how God could be acting in my life. After all, how could I be involved in an addiction that was so dangerous for so long? I had some questions and wanted proof that God was somehow involved in my daily personal life.

Was I being asked to surrender my will and my life, and give up my constant companion for something that is invisible? Was this just another authority figure trying to make me do what it wants?

Yes, I have questions, but when I accept that my old way hasn't worked, I can try new answers that have worked for others. I'm coming to believe that a Power greater than myself can restore me to sanity. This reveals a growing serenity and trust, because my Higher Power is in charge of guiding me from within.

Today, as I come to believe, build trust,
and get comfortable with my Higher Power,
my serenity grows.

FEBRUARY 23

You were sick, but now you're well again,
and there's work to do.
—Kurt Vonnegut

The way we join together to help each other in our recovery is what has made it possible for me to quit. I knew I could not do this alone. When I hit bottom, and pleaded with my Higher Power for help, I heard that small voice say "Get some support to quit smoking." I found online Nicotine Anonymous meetings and was encouraged by the people who were enjoying themselves before the meeting, laughing and having fun. This was so hopeful! These addicts were not using nicotine and were enjoying life.

At meetings I saw and heard that we are neither unique nor alone. Clearly, we share similar experiences with this addiction and obsession. We support each other and share a common hope.

Going to these meetings totally wrecked my smoking, and soon I was ready to begin the process of quitting. For me, meetings were my number one quit tool from NicA's Tools of recovery. Along with receiving unconditional help and support, I worked the first three Steps, did service work, reached out between meetings, and practiced the 5 Ds. All that helped me begin.

And the meetings, fellowship, camaraderie and friendships are what keep me coming back. I believe my Higher Power works through people in the program. I feel the comfort, safety, and the support offered by the fellowship. My job has been to be open to others' help.

Today, I allow others to help me.

Once the flood of emotions becomes manageable,
I find that life is a richer and swifter flowing stream.
I discover I can handle rough times. Time changes things.
Soon I find myself floating in moments of serenity.

—*A Year of Mracles*

When I was smoking, not only did I stuff my anger and fear, I stuffed my happiness and joy. In recovery, after allowing myself to feel a tiny bit of happiness and take it to heart, I wanted to enjoy it and not dismiss it. I could even share that happiness with others and that made the feeling grow.

I didn't have to be afraid or smoke over the feeling! Even as the happiness passed, I didn't sink down into the black hole of despair. I experimented with sadness and anger by allowing the feelings to just be what they were—feelings that come and go. As I work the Twelve Steps with my sponsor, I gain strength to believe in my ability to feel emotions with courage, rather than reacting with fear.

Doing the next right thing means that I ask my Higher Power and others for help in facing the big monster feelings I haven't dealt with yet. I avoid shrinking back and stuffing the feelings back down. The feelings begin to lose their power as I work the Steps and work through the feelings one by one—one day at a time.

*Today, I accept my feelings and allow them to flow
on down the river that is my life.*

FEBRUARY 25

We can only be said to be alive in those moments
when our hearts are conscious of our treasures.
—Thorton Wilder

Nicotine addiction can cause both physical and emotional heart disease. Denial disguised the pain enough so that I didn't recognize its glaring reality. However, my physical symptoms, news reports, and concerned family and friends all kept chipping away at the denial. Little by little, I acknowledged I had a problem.

Sometimes all I could do was nod my head, feel some shame, and then light up to console myself. I was in denial or just demoralized. It was difficult to have sweet moments, like when our hearts are conscious of our treasures.

The chemicals from nicotine not only deadened my senses but my heart's joy as well. This prevented me from truly celebrating my personal value. What I want from my recovery is conscious contact with who I really am and my personal treasures. As I come to believe in my authentic self, my sanity and serenity is restored.

The longer I live, the more I realize how short this precious moment of living is. In my spiritual practice, I humbly honor the treasures in each moment, which puts me more at ease with my mortality. I cannot change my mortality, but I can learn to celebrate my treasures during the time I have.

*Today, I live to engage in moments with my heart
fully aware of my value and my values.*

FEBRUARY 26

What I didn't have yet as courage,
I had as commitment to show up.
—Nicotine Anonymous Member

I stared through the window at a few people at a Nicotine Anonymous meeting. How could they possibly help me stop smoking? Convinced they weren't magicians, I drove home and inhaled even more nicotine. The next week, I entered and joined the meeting—my first surrender.

Despite my doubts, the members accepted me. I had a desire, but not yet the courage to stop smoking. Tradition Three says the desire to stop using nicotine is the only requirement for membership. That was comforting, but it also removed any excuse to escape.

Even with a book full of excuses for every situation in which I needed to get away with something, the groups' acceptance of me closed that book. I knew coming couldn't be a week-by-week decision because I would come up with a new excuse. I made a decision to commit and **Keep Showing Up**—my next surrender.

I didn't know how to stop smoking, so I did what I knew I could do—show up, share, and serve. Making that commitment, I became willing to go to any length. Eventually, I accepted **Lengths Become Strengths** and eventually I developed the courage to surrender nicotine. And so, I began my first of many more continuous 24 hours of being nicotine free.

Today, I am committed to show up, share, and serve—
grateful for my freedom, joy, and serenity.

FEBRUARY 27

Never say anything about yourself
you do not want to come true.
—Brian Tracy

For years I repeatedly said to myself, "I need a cigarette" or "I can't stop smoking." I learned in recovery that I come to believe what I continually tell my brain. My thoughts do not challenge such statements to realize they are lies. What my brain believes, I attract into my life.

Survival depends upon taking care of needs. By telling my brain, "I need a cigarette," my brain will relentlessly pressure me to satisfy that need until I act. Insanity is telling myself the life-threatening lie that nicotine is not lethal. When I tell my brain, "I can't stop smoking," my brain will agree and focus on what it can do and I light another cigarette. That's a familiar cycle, and the path of least resistance.

Now I mindfully notice the words I tell myself. The words in NicA literature are a good source of healthy thoughts and beliefs, especially hearing them read aloud. I need the sanity in those words. I go to meetings and hear what I need to live nicotine free. I come to believe those words, and my miracle comes true.

Today, I say the truth that sets me free.

FEBRUARY 28

There's no reason to smoke, it's only an excuse.
—Nicotine Anonymous Member

I came to meetings to be restored to sanity. It's true, I had no sane reason to smoke, only excuses. *Nicotine Anonymous: The Book*: says, "I had always thought of myself as fairly sane. But how could I have thought that when, forty or more times a day, I continued to smoke—when I knew it was killing me?"

I listened as members shared their truths. Without any criticism or unsolicited advice, there was no need to be defensive by shielding myself with excuses. We had a common problem, a common understanding, and a common solution—a spiritual program of recovery.

Meetings became my spiritual experience. Members' shares inspired me and filled my spirit with hope. Their honesty, openness, and willingness inspired me to transcend my excuses. They became my reason to sincerely work the Steps and use the Tools of recovery. Witnessing others' success at gaining freedom was a clear reason to accept that it works if you work it, and we are all worth it.

These are reasons why I came to believe that committing to a spiritual program of recovery, with no excuses, could make possible what I had thought was impossible and be restored to sanity.

Today, I have reason to believe.

FEBRUARY 29

He who cannot dance puts the blame on the floor.

—Hindu Proverb

Although I can hear music, I wasn't born knowing the steps to dance to it. To experience the joys of dance requires learning the steps and then practicing them. Likewise, quitting the use of nicotine is not something I innately know how to do.

Now in meetings, I hear that living nicotine-free requires the willingness to practice new behaviors. What I had been doing hadn't worked. Without the Tools of recovery to help, I am faced with repeated relapses. Failure tempted me to cast the blame at something else. Using blame to explain offers only excuses, not solutions.

Can I admit the reality that I, like millions of others, am powerless to control the craving for nicotine? This is a gentle way of accepting the responsibility without being "at fault." This leads me to seek the help in Step Two, rather than focus on what to blame.

As I learn the Steps for this dance, I can enjoy the music. I move more freely in the life that my Higher Power offers me. I find more than just a way to stop using nicotine. I discover a process that enhances my relationship with myself, with others, and with the Divine Creative Spirit of Life that conducts the music.

Today, I discover and practice the solution,
no excuses or blame.

MARCH 1

Made a decision to turn our will and our lives
over to the care of God *as we understood Him.*

—Step Three

When I first heard Step Three, I couldn't imagine giving up control like that. What would life be like? Wouldn't everything just fall apart without my managing things?

Starting with baby steps, I asked for the willingness to attend Nicotine Anonymous meetings and to really listen to what members were saying. I began to believe that even though I hadn't been able to quit on my own, a Higher Power could help me if I stopped trying to take control.

After months of meetings and failed attempts to quit, I was so demoralized I completely surrendered and gave my addiction to the God of my understanding. Then the miracle happened. The next day I woke up and didn't smoke. All day I didn't smoke. The next day too. Before long I had weeks, then months, and now many years without using any nicotine.

Clearly, Step Three has actually worked. Once I made the decision to turn my will and my life over to the care of God, my life started improving. First with smoking, then with everything else – my work, my family, my friendships, everything. My Higher Power used my addiction to shake me awake and show me a better way to live.

Today, I pray for the willingness to turn my will and my life over to a Power greater than myself, knowing that only good will come.

MARCH 2

I've found it's not my job to be in management, it's in labor.
—Nicotine Anonymous Member

If I was going to stop smoking, I would have to reduce my daily stress. In business, I was in charge. My job was the manager and "fix-it guy." Yet, I was so stressed I could not manage to stop smoking.

I found a NicA meeting where members recited the Serenity Prayer and closed with, "It works if you work it." In the pamphlet, "The Serenity Prayer for Nicotine Users," I was struck by the words, "Remember, it is not really the stress, frustration, or even the craving that causes us to keep using nicotine again, but rather our lack of serenity and courage to deal with the craving."

I bought *Nicotine Anonymous: The Book* and read sections on Steps One, Two and Three. I got Step One. Yes, I also needed sanity restored. In Step Three it said, "We needed to decide that we were no longer in charge and that we needed help." Hmmm, I needed help, but could I give up not being in charge?

So, my job in recovery is in the labor sector. My task is to work the Steps, and ask my new divine Manager for the serenity, acceptance, courage, and wisdom that restores me to sanity.

Today, I do the work and seek the courage
to change the things I can.

MARCH 3

The moment of surrender is not when life is over,
it's when it begins.
—Marianne Williamson

I lifted my eyes from staring at the meeting table when I heard a member share that she asked for mercy to relieve her of the bondage to nicotine. Mercy, a nicotine addict could ask for mercy? My shame had me feeling I did not deserve mercy, and so I did not think I could ask for it.

I came to realize my self-shaming led me to self-pity, and making excuses for my compulsive use of nicotine. When I needed self-care, I generally comforted myself with self-pity and nicotine. I wanted to change and do better, but alas, woe is me. And the cycle continued.

Indulging in self-pity until I finally surrendered, I asked my Higher Power for mercy and accepted grace. I became grateful that NicA is a gentle program shown by acceptance from my group. Easing my self-shame, I surrendered to a caring connection with the group. A sense of grace surrounded me like a soft blanket.

As suggested, I kept reciting lines from "The Serenity Prayer for Nicotine Users." As I read it over and over, I came to believe that the power we actually want is love! I found mercy and loving surrender in NicA.

Today, I humbly ask for mercy and offer support to others who seek the same peace that I seek.

MARCH 4

Oh yeah, I was willing to do the Third Step,
but I wasn't willing to turn over my cigarettes.
—Nicotine Anonymous Member

Although nicotine was probably my first drug addiction, it was the last to go. I thought putting down my other drug of choice was hard, but nicotine was the toughest.

To become willing to live without nicotine is a huge leap of faith, even for a veteran of another program. I already had come to believe in a Higher Power and had made a decision to turn my will and life over, but I kept making excuses to hold onto the nicotine. Exchanging my nicotine delivery device for the spiritual care of a Higher Power was a tough deal to make.

This is why it is important for me to have a fellowship that focuses specifically on nicotine, so I can learn to apply the Steps to this insidious addiction. Still, it took a bunch of Nicotine Anonymous meetings for me to have a breakthrough and surrender on a deeper level than ever before. Once I truly accepted that my ego could not control my use of nicotine, I began asking for help. As I became willing to receive my Higher Power's care instead of nicotine's toxicity, I began to let go of the clenching fear and resistance. That is when living without nicotine became possible.

Today, I surrender my diseased body and mind to spiritual care.

MARCH 5

We lost our best friend.

—Nicotine Anonymous: The Book

I came to realize I only *believed* I had lost my best friend. Nicotine appeared to work for a time, but when it stopped working, I didn't know how to do anything else. I was enmeshed in denial and nicotine's ability to alter my perception of reality.

My mid-life crisis was about facing increasing health consequences and an inner truth that kept breaking down my denial. I was in a battle between the nicotine nags and the truth tugs. Yet, I couldn't imagine how I could cope without nicotine.

No wonder, I hadn't developed much of anything else to actually manage my life, especially my emotions. Truth be told, nicotine was merely my best escape. Without nicotine, I had nothing to grab onto and nowhere to run.

Thankfully, I found a Nicotine Anonymous group. There were Steps, Tools, and the shared experiences from fellow addicts. I had a place to go. I became willing to practice doing what had worked for so many others. Now I have been restored to sanity with new behaviors to manage and enjoy my life.

Today, I practice what works because I am truly worth it.

MARCH 6

Sanity would suggest that our Higher Power's will for us
is to make life-affirming decisions
such as those that keep us free of nicotine.

—Nicotine Anonymous Step Study Workbook

Until recently, I couldn't understand on a practical level how I could decide to turn my life and my will over to the God of my understanding. Actually, all I have to do is be willing to have this Power greater than me be in charge.

I am not giving my Higher Power all my problems, I am simply willing to receive help and guidance. When I am struggling with self-will, I see that not turning something over to God IS self- will. Then clearly, I have more work to do in Step Three.

To begin getting some time free of nicotine, I started praying. I asked my Higher Power to help me accept and release my craving in the present moment, and to do what is suggested.

The initial freedom from nicotine is an incredible life changing experience, because I am not responding to every craving with a cigarette. I follow suggestions and make a life-affirming decision to not put a cigarette in my mouth, one craving at a time. Then I do this for just one day at a time. My job is to support my quit, no matter what life throws at me. As I am willing to receive help and guidance, my life becomes more serene.

---

*Today, I make life-affirming decisions
and receive God's guidance in all areas of my life.*

MARCH 7

I asked the question, "When will I get help?"
The answer I got was, "As you are ready."
—Nicotine Anonymous Member

Getting to the point where I was ready to receive the kind of help I needed came as a result of a process. For me, this process began out of fear. After years of frustration with this addiction, painful physical ailments, such as depression and shortness of breath, were making their presence known. I didn't begin this recovery process with a smile and a pile of hope. More than from intellectual awareness, my motivation came from deep in my gut.

The First Step of this recovery program is to admit we have a problem which we cannot control. After months of attending meetings while still smoking, I fell to my knees coughing and gasping for air. At that low point, both figuratively and literally, I admitted to myself that I needed help. Being on my knees was the beginning for me to stand tall.

The Second Step is coming to believe there is the help I need. I needed to allow some power stronger and better than nicotine into my being, into my life. My NicA group had been listening to me for months. Once I made the decision to turn my will and my life over to a Power greater than me, I became ready and able to accept the care I needed.

Today, I receive help as I am willing to allow and accept help.

MARCH 8

Meditation leads us to become still, open, and receptive.
—Nicotine Anonymous: The Book

In a life that's filled with to-do lists, commitments, and sticky notes, I often find my mind racing. That's my life today. When I quit smoking, I found my mind stepped up a couple of gears in all of the above. Plus, I mixed in random and intense thoughts such as, "What have I gotten myself into this time!" or "I can't quit smoking, who are you trying to fool!" And of course, there is always, "I want a cigarette; I have to have a CIGARETTE RIGHT NOW!"

I do today what I did then. I find a quiet place, sit down, close my eyes and say, "Be still and know that I am God." Then I start taking long deep breaths. When I recognize intense thoughts invading my mind, I simply say two words, "God Is" with each breath. I find that when I have gained a certain level of quiet, the stress or obsession that had been dominating my mind has passed. At that point I ask, "God what would you have me do next?" Most often the answer becomes clear to me. These mini-meditations help me through my day and focus with intention.

Today, I continue to improve my conscious contact with God for the peace that I seek.

MARCH 9

What would life be if we had no courage to attempt anything?
—Vincent Van Gogh

As a nicotine addict, the courage to change what had been familiar was very challenging for me. I looked to maintain my behavior so there would be a consistent and uninterrupted supply of nicotine. Any change was a threat. Any attempt to step out of my routine risked fear and failure. I did not want to rock the boat. My addiction was determined to stay afloat as if it were carrying me.

The anticipation of letting go of my drug was very frightening. For years, I had wished for the courage to face it. Now I am learning to ask for help from a Power greater than myself. At a Nicotine Anonymous meeting I heard, "Courage is fear that has said its prayers." I found that courage, like faith, needs to be exercised to get stronger. Now that I have found a source of courage, I need to use it, so I don't lose it.

Every day provides me with the opportunity to use my courage. I attempt new things and know the excitement of discovery. I enjoy this and am encouraged to keep up the momentum. I am doing what needs to be done: the next right thing. Recovery has shown me that sometimes I need courage to change things, and other times I need the courage to let them be as they are.

Today, I am grateful to have a source of courage
that helps me do what I once thought I could never do.

MARCH 10

Through surrender came the willingness to try anything,
including letting ourselves be helped
by something good and wonderful.
—Nicotine Anonymous: The Book

Surrender was necessary for me before I became willing to go even one day without nicotine. Then I found out that I had to surrender on a daily basis, and consciously make the decision to turn my life and will over to the care of God as I understood Him. *Daily basis* are the key words, because I truly can only remain nicotine-free one day at a time.

On days which are emotionally trying, I might find it necessary to pray the Third Step Prayer several times. I have heard people in the rooms say, "More will be revealed."

For me, that means that each time I read the literature, work on a Step or hear another member share his or her experience, strength, and hope, I find a more profound understanding of something good and wonderful.

I have to keep Steps One and Two in the forefront of my consciousness in order to thoroughly work Step Three. I can't, He can, I think I'll let Him. These Steps build upon each other, work together, and are a path to a spiritual way of thinking. I am learning from my fellow NicA members how to apply them. I continue to learn and practice the principles of our Program so I don't pick up.

Today, I surrender to the good and wonderful
God of my understanding to help me work the Steps
and stay free of nicotine.

MARCH 11

I don't get it. How can these Steps help me stop smoking?
—Newcomer in Nicotine Anonymous

At first, I wondered how the Twelve Steps could help me stop using nicotine. After years of addiction, I had a lot of doubt. I doubted myself and whether there could be anything that could stop this insidious and relentless urge to use nicotine. From years of experience, I came to believe that quick chemical solutions solved my problems.

My addictive mind welcomed doubt because it justified inaction. My mind wanted tangible proof before I even considered doing anything. When I was offered help, I looked for the program's flaws so that I could turn it down with good reasons. I was always looking for reasons to support my excuses.

Then I read the pamphlet, "How Nicotine Anonymous Works: Honesty Openness Willingness." I felt welcome among those who have gone before me and felt hope that there was a way to stop. I became willing to **Keep Showing Up**. I had to attend many meetings before my mind was willing to get that working the Steps could help me stop smoking. Eventually, the Steps got me, and I got quit.

Today, I get it, and use the Steps,
I am honest, open-minded, and willing.

MARCH 12

The power we actually want is love!
—"The Serenity Prayer for Nicotine Users"

Aw shucks. It's all about love. Members of my group loved me when I could not love myself. And then they showed me the Steps to recovery and the HOW of the program: Honesty, Openness, and Willingness. Now I'm learning to love myself, because members modeled that to truly love others, I must love myself first.

I believe my Higher Power loves me unconditionally, and wants the greatest good for me. I believe, no matter what, I cannot fail. I believe in the goodness of life.

Because I took the risk and allowed my fellow NicA members to love and help me through the process of quitting the insanity of the addiction, I have been shown a spiritual path and developed a relationship with a Power greater than myself. This relationship, and participation in my own recovery, gives me the courage to face life with openness, and trust that no matter what, all is well.

It's okay to try new activities and meet new people. There's a whole world out there to explore, enjoy, and feel good, because I don't need nicotine to face life or insulate me from love anymore.

Today, show me the way of patience, tolerance,
kindliness, and love.

MARCH 13

Keep me alert with courage to face life
and not withdraw from it,
not to insulate myself from all pain
whereby I insulate myself from love as well.
—Third Step Prayer

For the last 20 years of the 30 years I used nicotine, I wanted to quit. But whenever I ran out of my drug of choice and had to wait until I could get more, the withdrawal symptoms were miserable and deterred any hope of quitting. When I got more nicotine, there was temporary relief, followed by feeling miserable that I wasn't free of this madness.

If I'm going to be miserable anyway, better to be miserable moving forward toward freedom's relief rather than being miserable, stuck in the pain of addiction. When I found a NicA meeting with its program and Tools, I found a path to freedom. I had guide rails and hands to hold to support my journey from the misery of addiction to the relief of freedom.

I endured the discomfort of withdrawal, because I did not insulate myself from my fellow members' love and support. Members showed me their courage and inspired me to move forward, to accept the withdrawal, and know that I wasn't alone.

Today, I choose the relief of freedom,
through support, love, and courage.

MARCH 14

When the sun is not in the sky, then one sees the stars.
—Pir Vilayat Inayat Khan

I am learning to live life on life's terms. There is a time for lightness and a time for darkness. In the past when I became troubled, my addiction was triggered into high gear. When I felt emptiness, I reached for nicotine to fill me. There was no real serenity, only deadness. Through the haze I could not see the gems of those gifts available to me.

Darkness encourages me to ask for help and guidance. This is a good skill for me to develop, especially as a recovering nicotine addict prone to isolate when troubled.

This recovery program shows me healthier ways of taking care of myself, ways that clear the air and uncover the truth about living life on life's terms. Now I see light, even in the dark. The literature, the Steps and Traditions, the phone/email lists, my sponsor, and my Higher Power are all stars that help guide me through the dark.

As I come to believe, I see my Higher Power as my North Star—a constant in the changing skies of my life.

Today, I move forward even during dark, troubled times.
My recovery program sheds light on solutions.

MARCH 15

Acceptance has relieved me
of my battles on so many fronts.
—Nicotine Anonymous Member

Initially, I considered acceptance a sign of weakness. As an active addict, getting enough was the focus of my body and mind. Yet the serenity I ask my Higher Power for has many benefits. With time and practice, a new strength comes from this calmness. The less I focus on the things I cannot change, the less frustrated I feel. The less I look for busy distractions, the less disconnected I feel. Being peaceful offers clarity of purpose and more efficient action.

With this serenity, I sense my connection to the natural world's beauty that surrounds me and its grand and beautiful design. I let go of battles which don't serve my higher purpose or my recovery.

The world becomes less threatening. I feel less inclined to push and shove to try and change it. With calmness, I am not always worrying about getting enough.

Accepting the things I cannot change gives me serenity. I can relax into a deep spiritual connection, especially when I am in nature. Nature has its own design, which has been evolving for eons. It's a grand design to behold—if I can just hold still long enough.

*Today, I connect to my peaceful place within,
and find acceptance and serenity.*

MARCH 16

I find faith as I discover gems,
even tucked away in tiny places, brief moments.

—A Year of Miracles

As a nicotine addict, I did not handle frustration very well at all. It is one of the big buttons that pushed me to use tobacco. Unfulfilled desires are a lot of the heavy baggage I carried through life. When I chose nicotine as a means to ease the pain of my frustrations, I bypassed learning the life skills to deal with my feelings, which could have helped me become a more mature adult.

In recovery, I see that when I had been smoking, nicotine did not fix my frustrations, it increased them. Addiction is a cycle of insanity. I wanted to achieve a healthy, serene, and abundant life, but I was narrowly focusing in all the wrong places, over and over again.

As I practice the Third Step and place my life and will in the gentle care of a Power greater than me, my mind gets clearer about what really are the important things to obtain. As I turn my life over and trust a higher wisdom, I develop faith. Faith is a power beyond my rational thoughts—it comes from a conscious choice to focus on the voice of the heart rather than the intellect. Faith opens me up to the present moment, for the gems of contentment and fulfillment.

Today, I build faith on the gems that offer
a healthy, serene, and contented state of being.

MARCH 17

Be patient. Trust in God's timing. It's not that it'll never happen,
it just hasn't happened yet.

—Anonymous

To allow myself to even have the willingness to be willing to trust is the most enormous step I take as a nicotine addict. I allow my heart to open to the possibility of being happy, joyous, and free of nicotine. By practicing the principles of the program, I begin to trust the process of recovery.

Thank you Nicotine Anonymous for the experience, strength, and hope of those who have gone before us. Because those in recovery **Keep Showing Up** and doing service, they model a lifelong commitment to get and stay free from nicotine's powerful grasp.

Now, I allow my great creator to guide me to do the next right thing, to get myself to a meeting, and to participate in my own recovery process along this spiritual journey. I trust in my Higher Power's timing, and all is well.

Today, I allow my HP's will to unfold in my life,
and trust that the process is happening just as it should.

MARCH 18

To our great surprise we found that our decision
to surrender our will, and our willingness
to ask for help from a Higher Power,
or even from our fellow human beings,
was a liberating experience.
—Nicotine Anonymous: The Book

An addictions counselor once told me, "You have to surrender in order to win." I remember thinking that sounded crazy, but now I know it's one of those paradoxes of recovery. The only way I could "win" against my nicotine addiction was to give up, surrender, cry "uncle." Once I did that, my Higher Power stepped in and rescued me from its clutches.

It's a simple truth, but it took me a long time to comprehend. I kept trying this or that technique—switching brands, cutting back (fat chance), nicotine replacements—on and on, trying to fight my way to freedom.

None of it worked. It was only when I quit trying, gave up in utter defeat, that I finally got freedom. With that surrender, I got out of the way and my Higher Power did for me what I could not do for myself.

---

*Today, I surrender to a Power greater than myself
and trust that all is well in more ways than I can ever imagine.*

MARCH 19

Worry never robs tomorrow of its sorrow,
it only saps today of its joy.
—Leo Buscaglia

I spent years using nicotine while worrying about the consequences. Worrying kept me spinning around going nowhere. The more I wrestled with my worries, the more I numbed those worries with another hit of nicotine. Regardless of the delivery device, I stuffed emotions in an attempt to control them.

At my first Nicotine Anonymous meeting, we read about Step One. The sentence that jumped out was, "We learned about turning the tables, surrendering, and admitting our powerlessness." Surrendering? Well, my worry-wrestling had been a losing battle. The more I resisted, my fears grew, and the more intense they became. Relying on my own willpower was never enough to stop the insanity described in Step Two.

Step Three's reading said, "...asking for help was an act of strength, not weakness." I needed to surrender my struggle and become willing to accept a *greater care.*

I witnessed others' success using the Serenity Prayer instead of nicotine. They were learning the difference between what to accept and when to act. The NicA members in my group are my role models. They've helped me stop whirling around and turned me toward a greater power that works for me when I ask. I'm making progress, one surrender at a time.

Today, I am inspired by our slogan, ***Choose Faith Over Fear****,*
as I rise to life's occasions rather than worrying about them.

MARCH 20

As a nicotine addict, I wasn't afraid of dying,
I was afraid of living.
—Nicotine Anonymous Member

This boy could never be tough enough or safe enough among peers. That led me to believe I could fill what was missing in me with the promises of nicotine advertising and portrayals on a screen. Those adults appeared to be without fear and tough enough for anything.

The addiction became an obsessive need for nicotine that obliterated rational reasoning and defied reality. My attempts at numbing with nicotine led to a dumbing of my mind. I thought to be tough enough meant I had to ignore all threats of disease and death. I believed I couldn't survive living without nicotine as my shield. I got older, but stayed stuck in my immaturity with my secretive fears of inadequacy, trying to avoid the inevitable emotional pains of life. Ultimately, there wasn't a deadening of pain, just a dead end—the stark wall of what was still missing.

Our Third Step Prayer asks, "Keep me alert with courage to face life and not withdraw from it, not to insulate myself from all pain whereby I insulate myself from love as well." I came to believe I needed a spiritual power to grant me what I've been missing. For this day, I have enough and I am enough.

Today, I pray to my unconditional source with gratitude for doing for me what I could not do for myself.

MARCH 21

The most beautiful adventures are not those we go to seek.
—Robert Louis Stevenson

In the past I sought solutions by asserting my willpower. I barricaded myself behind my ego's pride. I was convinced that alone, I should determine my destiny. As an addict, I wanted complete control.

If I decided that the answer was off to the left, I was determined to go left. If life moved me to the right, I pushed back towards the left. I thought, "That looks so good over there, that's what I want, I must have that." Then came the frustration of failure, the pain from which I would plead, "What did I do wrong?" or "Why can't I have _____?"

The recovery process is, in part, a mysterious journey. I am not in complete control of when or how it will unfold. My work is to become willing and prepared to travel the path; spiritual principles will guide the way. I make plans for what I want, and as I make a decision to turn my will and my life over to the care of a Power greater than myself, I allow that Power to guide me.

With surrender, I discover paths previously unseen or unwilling to accept. As I entrust my faith in a Higher Power, I experience the peace, guidance, and care I have sought for so long.

Today, I follow my faith, that I may more fully enjoy the unfolding adventures of living.

MARCH 22

God can be an inner voice, nature,
other people, or a rock.
—Nicotine Anonymous: The Book

As I worked the first three Steps, I could turn my thoughts over, but I wasn't clear or convinced yet as to who or what I would turn them over to. I heard similar struggles with members trying to come to terms with Step Three. At first I struggled, because I've never been affiliated with any religious organization. My father enjoyed singing in church choirs. My mother was a member of a universal spiritual tradition. Their mission was to carry the message of spiritual common ground and the connection among all religions. I've always preferred developing my own personal path.

I have an idealistic streak, but appreciate what's practical, what works. I have come to believe a Power greater than myself can be my NicA group, nature's beauty, a Higher Purpose or Principle, among other inspiring concepts. Each concept provides what I want and need at the time. This works for me.

If I have a moment when I'm not feeling able to make conscious contact with someone or something specific, my first response is to be willing to let go of whatever it is that I need to turn over. I do this whether or not I have a spiritual presence to receive my will at that moment. If I'm troubled by something I cannot change and I'm unsure who or what to turn it over to, I'm comfortable turning things over to The Mystery.

---

*Today, I turn over my life's purpose
to a spiritual presence of my choosing.*

MARCH 23

My life was unmanageable because
I wasn't being a manager.
—Nicotine Anonymous Member

As an adolescent, I didn't start out prepared with a life plan. Without much of a clue, I had to get through my days by being clever and sneaky. My earliest capers were finding devious ways to get or steal nicotine. Those successful missions felt empowering and relieved some of my general anxiety and feelings of inadequacy. Having my chew tin in my shirt pocket was like wearing a sign, "That's right, I'm tough." I also discovered that nicotine's purpose was to medicate or numb my teen angst.

I didn't have much in the way of sensible life skills. I simply reacted to the moment, winging it as I reached for my constant companion in nicotine. I recklessly managed my daily interactions with life's situations. Nicotine was my short cut solution to every problem and accentuated every success.

Recovery has revealed that nicotine short-circuited my emotional process. As our Third Step Prayer points out, I may have insulated myself from all pain, but I also insulated myself from love as well. Life lessons to learn maturity were cut short. Turning my life over to this program with acceptance and courage has provided a path to stop being a reactor and instead become a wise manager of the life I want.

Today, I respond to life sensibly, without nicotine.

MARCH 24

Through trust in our Higher Power, we found that we were taken care of in surprising and simple ways.
Nicotine Anonymous: The Book

My life's experiences had shown me that people can't always be trusted to treat me fairly. I had long sought a lasting caring relationship, but the relationships were only temporary. Through those years, cigarettes were my consistent source of comfort and care, my trusted daily companions. That illusion lasted until the toxins took their toll and warning bells went off.

When I heard of a local NicA group, I decided to become a member. Yet, I resisted Step Three because my initial interpretation was that I should submit to a god I knew only others believed in. However, I became willing to turn a part of my life over to serving my group and fellowship. Eventually, I realized the essential word for me to focus on in Step Three was care. Care is what I had sought and no amount of nicotine was ever enough because it wasn't real care.

Time in recovery has helped me have lasting and caring relationships. Meetings have inspired my ability to exchange care through service and sponsorship. And this exchange has resulted in a spiritual connection to a greater care and a greater purpose. I trust in the power of this fellowship to heal and provide a care that I need and the peace that I seek.

Today, I allow something kind and powerful to care for me in surprising and simple ways.

MARCH 25

...Letting ourselves be helped by
something good and wonderful...
—Nicotine Anonymous: The Book

When I came to Nicotine Anonymous, I had a Higher Power I called God, but I thought He was too busy with real suffering to help me with my problem of nicotine addiction. However, after many relapses and many examples of others turning to their Higher Powers, I decided to let God provide "something good and wonderful," to come into my life. I quit with the thought that I would never again turn to a cigarette for comfort; I would only turn to God.

Ninety days into my quit, I was diagnosed with breast cancer. I prayed. I felt a hand touch my shoulder. "You will be okay," it was saying. I didn't light up. I really didn't care that I had breast cancer; I was overwhelmed with a new peaceful kind of joy. I was no longer a slave to the reactivity and urgency of addiction; I had allowed something good and wonderful to come into my life.

Today, I know in my heart that no matter what I am facing,
I have something good and wonderful
to help me through and keep me nicotine-free.

MARCH 26

Our concept of a Higher Power
will likely face challenges and changes over time.
However, this caring connection evolves
to provide a sense of peace and serenity.
—Nicotine Anonymous Step Study Workbook

My sponsor asked me to describe my Higher Power. "My HP is most kind and comforting, like wafting into soft pillows. As the ultimate life source, my Great Creator knows no limits and offers ever-continuous abundance. My Divine Light is the spark of life within me that connects all living things."

I've called my HP a variety of names and words like Source Energy, Universe, Divine Spirit, God, Light, Love, or Consciousness. The more expansive and inclusive ideas I have about a Power greater than myself, the more I connect with my very own version of the Great Spirit.

In Step Three I practice turning my will and life over to the care of this Universal Life Force. Praying, I ask for Source Energy's will in my life. Meditating, I listen. Very simple.

Happily, this is a program of progress not perfection. I make lots of mistakes, learn lessons, and give myself the grace to be a spiritual being having a human experience. I'm responsible for my reaction to life's situations. Where do I really want to focus my energy? Imprisoned by nicotine addiction?

I'd rather have peace and serenity. I'd rather be happy, joyous, and free. I can be through a conscious contact with the God of my own understanding, and by seeking my Divine Spirit's will for me.

Today, I ask for the willingness to trust, listen for,
and practice the Universe's will for me.

MARCH 27

I went for a walk in the woods, because trees inspire me
to look up rather than light up.
—Nicotine Anonymous Member

For years, I desired to live free of nicotine. I needed more inspiration than what I had during those times. Putting toxic chemicals into my body, one after another, was so incompatible with my beliefs of the natural world's boundless beauty and inherent integrity—all of which were designed to thrive.

Yet, on my own, I still couldn't, or wouldn't, overcome the fear that I couldn't manage my life without nicotine. I couldn't even imagine it. Meanwhile, the noxious substance and toxic shame continually eroded my self-esteem and spirituality.

When I joined a NicA meeting and read the pamphlet, "Our Policy of Openness," I found a fellowship where I belonged. I appreciated the acceptance and diverse beliefs about spirituality. Rather than diminishing my spirituality, this fellowship strengthened it. I had a place and people where I could express and explore my beliefs, and realize an emotional and physical benefit. At last, I had freedom to thrive!

I came to accept ownership and responsibility for my beliefs. This led me to turn over my belief that it was impossible for me to function without nicotine, and exchange it for the belief that it is possible. I can now live in harmony with nature's intention for me.

Today, I connect with nature's abundance
and let my spirit be lifted.

MARCH 28

Working Step Three has been all about
surrender and acceptance.
—Nicotine Anonymous Member

Making that decision has helped me realize that in any given situation, I am either in resistance to something or in acceptance of it. If I am in resistance, it's likely due to fear. Struggling against the current, I am suffering, which leads me back to nicotine.

When I am in acceptance, I am in the flow of my Higher Power's will and moving effortlessly through life with a sense of peace and openness. It is here that I feel most inspired and connected, and without the need for any crutch.

To get to a place of acceptance, I must consciously engage in a daily spiritual practice and constantly surrender. I say a prayer, often multiple times a day. In an instant, I am realigned with the feeling of love and connectedness I always longed for when I used nicotine.

While living life on life's terms, I consistently do a spot check of my feelings, followed by surrender and acceptance. Any cravings for nicotine subside. This is my ultimate defense against the cravings, and the resistance to acceptance that causes them. I turn over all of my resistance, negative emotions, and fears to my Higher Power.

Today, I choose to get out of my own way
and let my Higher Power take the lead.

MARCH 29

The tremor of awe is the best in man.
—Johann Wolfgang von Goethe

Being in a state of awe can be my most empowering experience and most humbling. I become right sized, and see myself in relation to my Higher Power even with fear haunting in the shadows. Recovery has helped me accept those scary feelings as just part of being human.

When I went to my first Nicotine Anonymous World Services Conference, I was both awed and frightened. I was amazed by others' courage to step up and serve the World Services fellowship, but I felt fearful about doing service myself. Eventually the awe that attracted me was greater than the fear that hindered me.

My smallness is humbling, yet somehow, I feel connected to the immensity. I have long been awed by the beauty of nature and the change of the seasons. I get goose bumps gazing up into the night sky dazzling with stars so far away. Those experiences helped me find the courage to offer service to the fellowship in World Services, a whole recovery universe beyond my local group.

Large and small awe-inspiring miracles happen to me and members of this fellowship. The miracle for me is my deep connection to this source of Power greater than myself.

Today, I experience awe with humility as I fulfill a higher purpose.

MARCH 30

Breathing is like ethereal drinking.
It is a luxury simply to exist.
—Henry Ward Beecher

I thought I really craved to inhale smoke. It seemed more important than anything. But would my priorities shift if suddenly I could barely breathe in any air at all? That would cause a real craving—for air!

The problem with smoking is that it didn't suddenly prevent me from breathing. It slowly crept up on me with a cough, then a wheeze. Then there was no glamour, no cool, just a gasp for air, and finally a willingness to seek help.

Fortunately, I learned about a local Nicotine Anonymous meeting, and was welcomed. I came to believe in the spirit of the group and breathed it in. Over time I got a quit going, returned to my senses, and only inhaled fresh air.

Breathing is my intimate connection with the outer world. It is a continual and constant resource. Without it, my lungs are empty, my heart has nothing to offer, and my brain is unable to think. Air offers the gift of life, and breathing is how I receive it.

Today, I step outside to take a deep, long moment of pleasure, breathing in presence.

MARCH 31

Free me from fantasy and fear.
—Third Step Prayer

Before becoming a NicA member, my head was filled with fantasy and fear, especially about my nicotine use. I fantasized about an effortless quit, and feared the pain of withdrawal.

I had fantasies of being superhuman, impervious to diseases from using nicotine. However, I believed I would quit if ever a doctor told me I had a dangerous condition. At the same time, I feared I could not live without my nicotine. All those fantasies and fears only built up my denial, and ultimately proved to be false.

"The Serenity Prayer for Nicotine Users" pamphlet says, "We kept hoping that in some magic way a day would arrive when the craving would disappear or we would find an absolutely painless way to stop being addicted. That day never came."

I found the magic elixir in Nicotine Anonymous. At first, I fantasized about having a stunt double and becoming two people: a smoker and nonsmoker at the same time. Others smiled as they had experienced similar flights of insanity. My fellow members' mutual understanding and support revealed a Power greater than myself that could restore me to sanity and freedom from nicotine.

Today, my life is grounded in reality
and inspired beyond my wildest dreams.

APRIL 1

To rid myself of the brainwashing of this addiction,
I needed an honest, deep cleaning.
—Nicotine Anonymous Member

The more meetings I went to and the more I read NicA literature, the more I realized how much my nicotine addiction affected my thinking, my feelings, and my beliefs. Every neuron in my brain seemed attached to a nicotine molecule. For years, I wanted to escape, but I couldn't get away from my addiction. My life was truly unmanageable and was thoroughly controlled and affected by nicotine.

It took time before I was willing to work the Steps. In Step Three, I developed my own understanding of a caring Power greater than myself. I began to understand the wisdom of the Good Orderly Direction of the spiritual sequence in the Twelve Steps.

Working Step Three enabled me to gain courage and strength through my Higher Power, which I needed to do Step Four's searching and fearless moral inventory. When I finally started my Fourth Step, I asked for the honesty to go deep and lift out character traits I did not want to admit.

In our quest for nicotine freedom, "Our Promises" express, "What relief!" The same comes from the deep cleaning, from clearing the debris of the past to make way for the good in the present and all the good that's yet to come.

Today, I humbly do my part to get to the truth of my behavior and attitudes.

APRIL 2

But one of the hallmarks of emotional maturity
is to recognize the validity of multiple realities
and to understand that people
think, feel, and react differently.
— Harriet Lerner

Doing my Fourth Step inventory helps me get a clearer view of my shortcomings and my assets. I also see how I have short changed my life from its full potential.

Maybe I had been resentful because I felt misunderstood; my life had been all about me. Maybe other people could not read my smoke signals; shouldn't they be able to figure out what I need? Maybe I rarely communicated without being under the influence of nicotine; I pushed others away.

Using tobacco shrouded me with a numbing buffer zone. This is one of the ways that nicotine made my life unmanageable. It prevented me from having real intimate contact with either myself or other people. There was an illusion of safety, but the clouded messages kept creating confusing feelings.

As a recovering addict, I see that when I was smoking, I was controlling to what degree I kept my thoughts and feelings from fully expressing who I really am. Now I accept my feelings without stuffing or denying them. By working the Steps, I learn emotional maturity, how to accept my feelings and express them in a healthy way.

Today, I communicate clearly about what truly matters.
I express my feelings with emotional maturity,
while respecting my own and others' feelings.

APRIL 3

If every day I expand my belief
in the possibilities available to me,
imagine what wonderful things could happen.
—*A Year of Miracles*

I used nicotine to lessen my anxiety about being seen for the person I feared I was. I had a distorted view of who I feared I was and who I actually am. I behaved with an exaggerated dramatic flair to disguise the feeling of inadequacy that I feared people might see within me. I paraded about, with billows of smoke, to create an appearance of confidence. I adopted the persona of characters I saw on TV and in movies. With the numbing effects of nicotine, I didn't even care that I was living a charade.

Working the Twelve Steps offers me a way to see both character assets and how I can improve. The Steps are a guide out of the haze of addiction that shrouded my reality. The humility and honesty that recovery develops breaks down the ways I have betrayed myself and my beliefs. I forgive myself for letting fear determine my behavior. I accept and love myself for who I really am. I am enough.

Today, I accept all that I am
and all I want to become.

APRIL 4

Nodding the head does not row the boat.
—Irish Proverb

Step Three brought me to the place where I had to make a decision to turn my life, my will, and my smoking over to a Power greater than myself. Since I knew I was powerless, and everything was a power greater than me, it wasn't hard. But that decision had no impact on my life without taking action, which meant moving on to the next step.

Step Four was a bit scary, but I started, and it got easier. By the time I had finished, I had a tool for problem-solving in my life. With practice, Step Four has become a useful, simple tool I use again and again.

I use it even for simple things. For example, I moved to a new area, and I gave out my cell phone number to members of a service committee. I left my number and a message to call me, but nobody called me back. I developed a resentment. Then I knew I needed to work Step Four again.

What was my part? I realized that people in my new home region were not used to having to dial an area code. So, I got a new number with a local area code. And my phone started ringing. I am now happily engaged in service. Keeping the focus on me and my part, and doing the next right thing is recovery in action.

Today, I will remember to do the footwork
and leave the results to my Higher Power.

APRIL 5

I like criticism, but it must be my way.
—Mark Twain

Criticism is a behavior pattern I included in my Fourth Step inventory. To make decisions includes my intentions and requires discernment. Choices involve analyzing and evaluating situations. However, I have numbed my emotions and responded to making choices by using nicotine instead. Recovery means taking a close look at the intentions behind my choices.

I have been critical and judgmental of others' decisions in order to avoid looking at my own behavior. As an addict, I always came up with excuses for the way I acted. The cravings of my addiction created an urgent, needy self-centeredness. Both my unease and disease led me to be controlling; I wanted things my own way.

The wisdom of this program guides me to be more at ease with myself and with life on life's terms. I accept that I cannot always have things go my way. I realize that I am not wise enough to always know what is best for me.

I am coming to believe in a Higher Power to whom I can entrust my life. Although I still have to be discerning, I am now careful that any criticisms are not just cloaked excuses and distractions. With others' support and example, I seek to determine the truth about myself.

Today, I am guided. I make wise and honest choices.

APRIL 6

Every strike brings me closer to the next home run.
—Babe Ruth

Before I was a nicotine fiend, I was a baseball fan. As a kid we played stick ball in the street. By myself, I'd spend hours pitching a ball at a strike zone chalked on my school's wall. I became a Little League pitcher and struck out opponents with an accurate fast ball. As a batter, I had my share of strikeouts. My reassuring coach would say, "Keep swinging away." I still say that today when things don't work out at first.

Those words helped me through several strikeouts with relapses. I tried to switch hit with vaping, but that wasn't getting me on base. I remembered the key to my accurate pitching was to always follow through, so I kept showing up. As Yogi Berra said, "It ain't over 'til it's over."

I kept swinging away until I hit a home run, which I do every day I stay abstinent from nicotine. It took a team of Nicotine Anonymous members to help me hit nicotine out of the park and get free.

I'm grateful for the NicA meetings to return to each week. I have a safe place to be accepted and remain accountable for my actions. I'm staying in the game.

Today, with a spiritual coach, I step up to the plate to face whatever comes my way.

The shortest answer is doing.
—English Proverb

Before Nicotine Anonymous, the best I was willing to concede was "I will *try* to change, *try* to stop smoking." This was mainly a way to placate someone else's request or even my own. All too often, trying became a set up for not doing. By saying, "I'll try," I avoided admitting that I won't do it. It got me off the hook for the moment. But I was still hooked. *Trying* was just an excuse to escape the reality of my behavior. I sought comfort by saying, "Okay, I'll try."

I was not able to stop smoking when I started going to NicA meetings, but I became inspired by what members were *doing*. I began to ask myself, "Okay, what am I willing to do?" I learned, *doing is what gets it done.*

I accepted that I can go to meetings, read literature, make phone calls, pray, and do many other things that I have the power to accomplish. My focus could be on what I am willing and capable of *doing*. No matter how small the deed, action can be my answer to stop being stuck. Doing creates more doing.

Today, it feels good to be doing,
rather than making up another excuse.

APRIL 8

The only thing worse than being blind
is having sight but no vision.
—Helen Keller

Writing out my Fourth Step moral inventory revealed how I sought to take shortcuts or to get away with things. I'd been resistant and rebellious, arrogant, and defiant. Such traits once seemed necessary survival weapons, which I used due to my lack of developing more mature skills to manage my life.

Now I see how nicotine contributed to much of the chaos in my life. My addiction stifled my emotional and spiritual growth, my ability to see beyond the next hit. I lived in a drug-deluded state of mind. I thought my shortcomings served me.

I used the drug just to survive, not live. Since I wasn't prepared to deal with life's challenges, nicotine's effects reduced my ability to learn and change. To escape any discomfort or pain I would just light another cigarette, which fed many other bad habits in my attitude and behavior.

To recover and not relapse, I became willing, not resistant, humble, not arrogant. I learned to be patient with this process and myself. By working NicA's program of recovery, I am preparing myself for each day, both the good and the bad, and living life on life's terms. The truth is, I was blind, but today I can truly see.

Today, my faith gives me hope and a vision of the way forward.

APRIL 9

If we go down into ourselves,
we find that we possess
exactly what we desire.
—Simone Weil

To be alive and conscious is to desire. Beyond physical survival, I desire to know myself and the purpose for my being in this experience called life. I want to feel my connection with the cosmos, with something greater. I desire an inner peace and a spiritual connection to the whole, which has eluded me.

The desire to feel connected to others is part of human nature. I did a thorough search during my Fourth Step inventory, and realized how this desire has been involved in my misguided behavior to "fit in." Humility that comes from working the Steps creates a bridge that connects me to my Higher Power's guidance to fulfill a higher purpose, to find inner peace and a spiritual connection.

Possessions can be tools in my survival. They can even offer me comfort. However, the serenity I seek cannot be manufactured in a product or delivered by a drug. That serenity comes not from what I can hold in my hands, but what I can cherish in my heart. My heart constantly beats a calling, reminding me that the answer is within.

Today, the inner peace I desire is always within me.
Seeking my Higher Power's guidance,
I connect with my higher purpose.

APRIL 10

It always seems impossible until it's done.
—Nelson Mandela

For long years, my continual wish to stop imprisoning myself with nicotine was always crushed by my belief that freedom was impossible. Yet, Nelson Mandela's life journey is an inspiring example of perseverance —with moral principles intact—despite long imprisonment and solitary confinement.

By joining Nicotine Anonymous, I met many inspiring people from all over the world. I listened to their experience, strength, and hope from their perspective. Some were still in the struggle, like I was, but others were done using nicotine, one day at a time. They united in mutual support to gain and maintain freedom from the chains of this demoralizing addiction.

Their inspiration has been a spiritual experience. Their support encouraged me to do my own searching and fearless moral inventory. Then I better understood the concepts of Step One about how my nicotine use was a symptom that my life had long been out of control and unmanageable.

Our slogan, **Together We Change**, explains that unity is how my impossible becomes our possible. Together, with program principles, is how we get the impossible done.

Today, I stay connected with members
and focus on Nicotine Anonymous rather than nicotine.

APRIL 11

At a point in every person's life,
one has to look deeply into the mirror of one's soul
and decide one's unique truth in the world,
not as one may want to see it or hope to see it, but as it is.
—James McGreevey

When I first tried to stop smoking, I realized that stress wasn't the only factor for having a cigarette. I thought using nicotine right after having a good time was a choice I made, a pleasure I afforded myself. When attempting to quit, I discovered using nicotine after good times wasn't a choice, it was a compulsion. There was some emotional need that still made a cigarette seem necessary.

My Step work became a daring look deep into the mirror. As a nicotine user, I had stunted my emotional and spiritual development. Any amount of anything, even a good time, never felt like enough. Those moments after a good time had awkward pauses—with a nagging unsatisfied, unidentifiable emptiness, an inability to feel fulfilled and content. I believed that only nicotine could provide this fulfillment.

At meetings, Nicotine Anonymous principles guide members to create a safe place to interact without a smokescreen. I can be vulnerable, authentic and open to mutual support. I develop an ability for emotional and spiritual fulfillment. That's where and how I can get and can give enough. That's where I see my unique truth as it is and accept myself where I am.

Today, I share my life deeply and fully,
noticing and savoring the good moments.

APRIL 12

Integrity is telling myself the truth.
And honesty is telling the truth to other people.
—Spencer Johnson

We each have our own way of getting to the start of a quit and making it, one day at a time, through the cravings and into freedom. For me it took honesty with myself about the effects of nicotine on my body, mind, and spirit. Little by little, the recovery dialog began chipping away at ol' nicodemon's armor. Working the Steps, writing, reflecting honestly, and sharing in meetings slowly eroded the addiction's hold over me.

Other members' willingness increased my willingness to consider putting cigarettes down. Even before I quit, I was one of those addicts who was already disgusted by cigarettes, but NicA meetings lifted any notion about enjoying smoking. For me, that was the important chink in ol' nicodemon's armor. That thin slice of honesty began to expose my addiction. As the smokescreen lifted, I could clearly see the power nicotine had over me.

It takes a lot of courage to share honestly about what we are going through. Nicotine loses its power in the face of honesty, openness, and willingness.

Today, I am truthful and honest with myself and others.

APRIL 13

If I constrain my spirituality to being about me,
I rob us all of the richness we can experience
when united for a higher purpose.
—Sarah Bowen

I was self-centric. When I used nicotine, my behavior and attitude was so much about me and the drug I wanted. In my early years, I felt empowered because nothing could stop the power of my will to use. Eventually, as with most nicotine addicts, that behavior and attitude stopped working. I became enslaved.

I saw glimmers of maturity and began to face health issues in that self-reflective mirror of mid-life crisis, and it became clear that I had no power to stop using nicotine. I'd sadly stare at full ashtrays and see my ongoing legacy. Nicotine had been my reliable companion. Without my drug, it was only me, myself, and I.

At NicA meetings, I found new companions, my fellow nicotine addicts. I felt connected to their struggles and successes. When I finally turned my will over to a Power greater than myself, I became liberated from nicotine and wanted to inspire others. There was such richness to this human experience.

I accepted requests to serve, first locally, then at World Services. I collaborated with others to carry the message. Together, we've created a far better legacy than a pile of toxic ashes.

Today, I experience my spirituality
by uniting with others for a higher purpose.

APRIL 14

A man should live only to satisfy his curiosity.
—Yiddish Proverb

I was born curious. I was anxious to explore and determined to walk. I asked endless questions about everything around me. Curiosity continues to urge me past old limitations. It is a spice that adds zest to my journey. I am surrounded today with possibilities and pleasures invented by the curious.

However, since my teen years, my addiction to nicotine spread cynicism over my life. Nicotine deadened feelings and drained my enthusiasm. The cravings kept me chained to limits within reach of my pack. I wouldn't go where I couldn't smoke. I developed real physical limitations that kept me from exploring and playing.

When I heard about Nicotine Anonymous, I had just enough curiosity left to show up at a meeting. Listening to others helped stimulate my curiosity. I heard how they were using this program, not only to break the chains of nicotine addiction, but to explore the call of their curiosity and to consider their wildest dreams of possibilities. Yes, this was a recovery to boldly go where this nicotine addict would never have gone before.

Today, I honor my curiosity by stepping forward to discover more possibilities.

I had an "addiction-ary" filled with excuses and lies
that defined my behavior and attitude.
—Nicotine Anonymous Member

For me, my addiction-ary included excuses and lies such as, "I love to smoke," "cigarettes are my best friend," "smoking is my only vice," "I gotta have a crutch," "I need a cigarette," "everyone's gonna die someday from something," "someday I'll stop." Nicotine was the author and the task master that kept me believing these lies.

When a health crisis finally got me to go to a Nicotine Anonymous meeting, I listened to truths I recognized but had been too afraid to face before. I heard how other members turned over their lives to a Power greater than themselves to gain honesty, compassionate connection, and mutual support.

I exchanged my addiction-ary for NicA literature. I now had books of wisdom and guidance. I accepted the care offered. I began to reclaim my mind, heart, and soul. I can now redefine my life.

*Today, I experience the power of honesty,
compassionate connection, and mutual support.*

APRIL 16

Very often a change of self is needed
more than a change of scene.
—A.C. Benson

For years I took comfort with the illusion that I really didn't need to change and give up my nicotine habit. As my health began to deteriorate and my doctor said I needed to stop smoking, I responded with excuses. The time was "not right," and I had issues with where I lived and with my job. I thought I would have to wait until I could make changes in my life's situations before I could even consider quitting smoking.

I moved to a different area and got into a different type of work. My life was better in some ways, but I continued to smoke. That didn't change. When I started getting chest pains and a cough, I thought it was enough to switch to a light brand of nicotine. I bought the lie.

Eventually I had to admit that changing my outer world was, at best, only a temporary fix. When I discovered Nicotine Anonymous, I realized I needed an inside overhaul to be restored to sanity. At meetings I learned recovery begins from within. How the program works is with my honesty, open-mindedness, and willingness.

Today, it's an inside job for me to truly change my life and recover.

Step Four opened the door to secrets
I even kept from myself.
—Nicotine Anonymous Member

I wanted to stop using nicotine for years but did not and suffered with the shame of this failure. In my past I usually found ways to get away with things and take short cuts causing more pain. My sponsor suggested that in working Step Four, I look for any attachment to suffering. That seemed odd, but I was guided to make a thorough *searching and fearless moral inventory* of myself.

Change happens when a person finally reaches a physical, emotional, or spiritual bottom and surrenders to inevitable renewal. My Step work involved answering why I was enduring such suffering before I hit my bottom.

Did suffering give me permission to justify my defensive defects? Did it support my self-pity or my self-image as a victim? Did I need pain to permit myself to take care of myself without guilt? If I maintained suffering, did that allow me my pleasure of using nicotine? What secrets have I kept from myself? Now, I need to be willing to go to any length to discover answers about myself.

Today, I continue working a thorough Fourth Step to discover anything that stands between me and my joy.

APRIL 18

Success is a journey, not a destination.
The doing is often more important than the outcome.
—Arthur Ashe

For so many years I felt like I was not successful. I compared my financial career track with others and felt that I had less than they did. I achieved quite a few milestones, but still did not feel successful.

Now, I am an artist, a painter, which is my true-life purpose. As long as I am producing creatively, I am successful because I am listening with my heart more than my mind.

Spiritual fitness is one of my necessities on this journey. I require spiritual growth to maintain my freedom from nicotine. I grow spiritually when I help others. When I work the HOW of the program: Honesty, Openness and Willingness, I grow spiritually.

Success also means being true to myself. When I am honest about my abilities as well as my difficulties, I know what I have to work with. Once I was influenced by others' opinions, now, I am better off following my Higher Power's will for me. I trust myself to seek my HP's guidance, which I know in my heart I can trust.

Today, I seek success through the journey of the heart.

APRIL 19

If you have faith, then your whole life
is put in a new perspective.
You get to work but enjoy the work at the same time.
If you grow spiritually, you do what's in front of you
and let the results speak for themselves.
—Roy Orbison

Quitting is a process of learning what it is that makes me want to use nicotine. I spent many months trying to quit every single day. I based this on the illusion that The Magic Anti-Smoking Fairy would someday hit me on the head with its wand, and I would no longer smoke. Or maybe I was bound to make it if I just kept on trying. Sometimes I made it a few days, maybe a week, but I was never free of the addiction.

Once in Nicotine Anonymous, I learned why I was addicted to nicotine. I came to understand that smoking one cigarette is not just one hit of nicotine but provides multiple hits of the drug. Speaking to my NicA friends, I came to understand the addictive nature of smoking and how it imprisoned me in the addiction. Everything started to make sense.

Now, I cannot tolerate any nicotine, and am grateful for the gift of recovery our program offers. I work a few simple Steps and practice the principles of the program. As I grow along this spiritual path, I am amazed at how my mind has changed from wanting that hit, to no longer wanting to use. There was no magic fairy involved. I came out from behind the smokescreen to see the world in a whole new light.

Today, recovery is giving me the spiritual life I want,
and the results speak for themselves.

APRIL 20

Stay in the middle of the herd.
—Nicotine Anonymous Member

Craving, emotionality, and turmoil were a part of my life for so long. As I attended meetings, I began craving the relief of freedom from the insatiable nicotine monster.

By the time I quit, I had worked the first three Steps with my sponsor. It made all the difference that I had started building that relationship with a Power greater than me. Every time I craved, I asked my Higher Power to help me, and every time, HP helped. As the days passed, my relationship with HP grew and grew.

At one point early in my quit, I was so raw and emotional that I curled up under the covers, because that was all I could think of to do. I didn't light up. I wrapped my HP's arms around me for safety and comfort when the world seemed to be triggering my anger, emotionality, and stinking thinking. And the cravings passed.

Friends in NicA reminded me that smoking would not help my emotions, only stuff them back down. Smoking wouldn't solve any of the problems or character defects I was dealing with. Smoking only makes them worse.

I turned to my work in recovery, attended meetings, worked the Steps, did service work, read literature, and reached out for help. Today I still **Keep Showing Up**, because my HP, NicA friends, quit buddies, and sponsor, are all there for me.

Today, I support my recovery
and my new way of life.

APRIL 21

The truth is, no matter what your lifestyle or occupation,
nothing can really stop you when you're allowing yourself
to be exactly who you want to be.

—Hayley Williams

I pleaded with the Universe from the deep bottom I'd hit. My life was so excruciatingly unmanageable. I searched for help online. I found an online Nicotine Anonymous meeting that was about to start. The virtual meeting room had about 20 people who were laughing and joking around. Like friends, they were happy to see each other. These people were quitting using nicotine? I wanted what these people had!

My use of this drug had gotten so out of control that I was shut off from laughter, from goodness, from friends. I had no life except my addiction. I had no idea who I was or what I wanted anymore. I heard my Higher Power say, "Allow." I knew what this meant—to allow the goodness, to allow the process to unfold, to allow the strength of these people to help, to allow myself to trust this process.

As the members congratulated each other on their time free of nicotine, hope grew in my heart. Some had weeks, others months, even years. Something must be working here if these folks can celebrate their time free from this powerful addiction. When I introduced myself, I was applauded, congratulated, and warmly welcomed. All I had done was show up!

Today, I show up to allow myself to become
the person I really want to be.

APRIL 22

Nicotine is a mind-altering drug.
A relentless predator, it made my mind crave
endless amounts of nicotine.
—Nicotine Anonymous Member

I have a desire to stay off nicotine, but there is this nicodemon in my brain who has lived there for years and is angry at being evicted and punishes me with pain because I defy it. Even in recovery, nicodemon can still fog up my thoughts with all sorts of excuses to keep using the drug. My addiction has me resent others who are still using, even those in my group. I think, "How dare they trigger my cravings!" But this addiction is about me, not them.

My sponsor reminds me I am in a transition. My mind may be saner, but definitely still on its way to being restored to sanity. I may still find smoking scenes in movies alluring, smoke on the street aromatic, and resent others who smoke instead of being grateful I'm not. As an addict, I'm unaccustomed to waiting to be relieved of any discomfort.

This journey takes patience, commitment to practice principles, and the willingness to move toward a spiritual awakening. As my conscious contact grows, I transition from believing in nicodemon's lies to choosing the sanity of my Higher Power's grace and comfort.

Today, Higher Power, please lift me from the fog
and help me gain clarity.

I was still playing hide and seek,
with my Higher Power calling,
"Come out, come out wherever you are."
—Nicotine Anonymous Member

When I switched from smoking to vaping a nicotine concoction, I was still addicted and still attempting to live undercover, behind a cloud. I operated like a spy in my own life.

During my Fourth Step inventory, I became willing to write down my shames, fears, and feelings of inadequacies. I acknowledged that, as a child, I wanted to take on the identity of those people in advertising images. Whenever I was asked, "What do you want to be when you grow up?" I had no idea, except maybe one of those people in the glorified images. Then came vaping, and I accepted the illusion that it was safer and its technology made me look hip.

Answering questions in the *Nicotine Anonymous Step Study Workbook*, I began to come out of hiding and even learn good things about myself I didn't know I was hiding. At meetings, I also learned my secretive spy life is not unique and somewhat normal for a nicotine addict.

In NicA, I'm accepted for who I am, with all my flaws and strengths. Our book states, "We were not awful. We were humbled to realize that we were normal—and just very human." I'm retiring from the hide and seek game, one breath at a time.

Today, I have the courage to discover the good person I really am.

APRIL 24

You have been invited to the divine banquet,
and here you are crawling after crumbs.
—Pir Vilayat Inayat Khan

The Great Creative Spirit of the Universe presents me with such a bounty of things, experiences, and opportunities. True, not all of them arrive gift wrapped, or are what I really want. This is why I have hindsight.

All too often I had been willing to crawl after crumbs, settle for the least. While others feasted at the divine banquet, I sought comfort in less, so that I could avoid disappointment. Nicotine numbed me so early, I hadn't fully realized how good life could be. Thankfully, life is a process, so when I pay attention, wisdom comes with time.

Now, with the care of my Higher Power and sponsor, the insights I gain from doing my Fourth Step can inspire me to let go of my self-deprivation and to embrace the bounty of spiritual nourishment. Without burdening my body with nicotine, I have the energy to do enjoyable things that before I was not able to do or let myself have. As my ability and attitude improve, new opportunities open for me.

---

*Today, I receive the bounty
of my Higher Power's divine banquet.*

APRIL 25

Every experience, however bitter, has its lesson,
and to focus one's attention on the lesson
helps one overcome the bitterness.
—Edward Howard Griggs

As my days came and went, they arrived and left with assorted flavors. Some were quite bitter. Often it was my resistance to accepting the lesson I was being offered that caused the foul taste. When I was active in my addiction, I was not really looking for any lessons; I was too busy looking for another match.

Repressed anger in my childhood was part of the reason I first picked up cigarettes. For years I was too pissed off to care about any lessons. I didn't really want to behave any better.

Over time I came to realize that my attitude was not making my life better, which was a bitter pill to swallow. Reluctantly I joined a Nicotine Anonymous group. By observing my fellow members' examples, I discovered the sweet gifts of the lessons they teach. Our literature says I can be happy, joyous, and free. Just **Keep Showing Up**. It's a sweet deal.

Today, I accept the sweet serenity and courage
I gain from the valuable lessons I am learning.

APRIL 26

Using nicotine was more than a bad habit, rather,
it was a symptom that our lives
were out of control and unmanageable.

—Nicotine Anonymous: The Book

I've had a suitcase full of excuses that I've been traveling with for a long time. For years, one of the ways I tried to manage my life was with my multitude of excuses. Excuses appeared to help control things, especially to cover up my inadequacies and shortcomings. But I knew the excuses were mostly lies. My life had become a lie.

My Fourth Step work showed me that the control I sought was actually as flawed as the excuses. Excuses and lies just added to the things I needed to control. My shame over this behavior was alleviated when I was told I could forgive myself and ask for mercy from the grace of this gentle program.

With time in recovery, I have been granted the humility and courage to work on letting go of excuses and to simply focus on being honest, open, and willing to do the next right thing. I use the Steps and the Tools to help manage my daily activities. They work, and I have every reason to use them.

Today, I practice humility and courage to change myself.

Someday is not a day of the week

—Janet Dailey

I lost count of how many years I consoled myself with the lie, "Someday I'll stop smoking." Saying "someday" was one of many justifications I used to continue using nicotine. I was sweeping the truth under a cloud of smoke.

When we read Step Four at my Nicotine Anonymous meeting, I often got to read the sentence, "The important thing was to do it." I struggled with the fear of what I would face doing the Fourth Step work. I consoled myself by saying, "Someday I'll work on my Fourth Step."

I kept thinking that smoking was soothing my anxieties. But then, listening at meetings, I came to hear the truth, that using nicotine kept me continually anxious. I realized the excuses and lies I used were my attempts to soothe that anxiety. Self-soothing is a human need, but a key to recovery is developing healthy and sane ways to do that.

I finally surrendered my resistance and sought the courage to write answers in our *Nicotine Anonymous Step Study Workbook*. I surrendered my excuses and got a sponsor to discuss my responses. As the smoke cloud has cleared, my serenity grows, and I am becoming more honest and serene.

Today, I find comfort in healthy and sane ways of living as I seek the courage to change the things I can.

APRIL 28

People never believe in volcanoes until the lava overtakes them.
—George Santayana

I once had a friend who nagged me, telling me I was like a smoking volcano that would eventually erupt. Angry, I blew him off. My denial enabled me to delude myself into thinking that wouldn't happen to me. Somehow, I would be different, I was special. That was the kind of arrogant belief I had when I was using nicotine.

So, I denied the rumblings of the nicotine-related diseases that begin unnoticed inside and slowly build up. Eventually, these diseases overtake the body and offer little or no mercy. I dismissed the fact that millions of people die each year from smoking-related diseases. I ignored how others become ill or die from secondhand smoke.

Then, my mother's lung cancer snapped me out of denial. I found Nicotine Anonymous. Now, instead of erupting when others express their concern, I can tell them I'm on a path with a program to help me find freedom. That is why I work this program daily with the help of a Power greater than myself, my sponsor, and my friends in recovery. Now I listen, with humility, as others share their experience, strength, and hope. And I feel a new peace.

Today, I am grateful I belong to a fellowship that supports my new life free of nicotine.

APRIL 29

Your attitude, not your aptitude, will determine your altitude.
—Zig Ziglar

Once upon a time in my fantasy tale, I used an arrogant devil-may-care attitude to cover up feelings of inadequacy, like my inability to stop using nicotine. I would also seek comfort in cynicism and negativity to avoid anticipated disappointments. I displayed an attitude that I was somehow unique, and that I would not suffer any consequences due to smoking. But deep down, I really didn't believe that lie.

As I worked on my Fourth Step inventory, I admitted that many of the attitudes I displayed as external reactions were little more than a defense to cover up what I felt inside—thinking this was how I needed to manage my life. Now, I see that I created my own disharmony, a form of my insanity.

The Serenity Prayer helps me get clear so I can respond with wisdom, rather than react with a defensive coverup. I am not powerless over my attitudes. Guided also by the Third Step Prayer and program principles, I see how I create my own attitude and how I experience my interactions in my daily life. As I practice being more mindful of my attitudes and responses, I develop a new trust and confidence that I can manage whatever comes my way.

Today, I ask for the courage to change the things I can, especially my attitudes.

APRIL 30

The first step toward change is awareness.
The second step is acceptance.
—Nathaniel Branden

When I work Step Four, I work closely with my sponsor. My objective is to become aware of my assets and shortcomings, and share my findings with my sponsor.

As I work Step Five, my sponsor points out my character assets and the shortcomings that became the extreme behavior I used to get my needs met when I was younger. These behaviors no longer work for me today. There is no blame, but I am accountable for my actions.

I get to work on these shortcomings one by one. Step Six helps me become entirely ready to change, and then when taking Step Seven, to humbly ask God to remove these defects of character.

The simplicity of our program of recovery helps me to increase my awareness of how each defect's discomfort feels while I'm practicing it. I come closer to accepting the behavior and taking action to change that defect into an asset that works. This is how I find the peace and serenity I seek.

Today, I move from awareness to acceptance to action, giving myself kindness and care while doing my Step work.

MAY 1

Admitted to God, to ourselves, and another human being
the exact nature of our wrongs.
—Step Five

The Twelve Steps guide us to be thorough and sincere with powerful words such as admitted, decision, fearless, exact, entirely, promptly, conscious, and awakening. At first, I was intimidated and had defensive reactions. Yet, after so many failed attempts to quit, my powerlessness was undeniable. How could I not need help and care? I decided I had to **Keep Showing Up** at meetings.

My inventory included two main character defects I used to mismanage my life. I was adept at making up excuses and lies, and getting away with things. I needed to assess and testify to their exact nature and realize that they were morally wrong and perpetuated my addiction and its compulsive behaviors. This work on my defects brought me to surrender my defenses and own up to specific truths about myself. Despair gave way to hope. Stress gave way to serenity. Fear gave way to courage. Lies gave way to truths.

In recovery I learned to become honest, open, and willing. I often recite The Serenity Prayer. It is simple and easy to remember, but powerful. It directs me to seek wisdom and realize the difference between the value of truth and unmanageable lies. "Our Promises" are coming true for me, one day at a time.

Today, I prepare to be entirely ready to change the things I can with the care of a Higher Power and guidance of this program.

MAY 2

Talking to you is only thinking to myself—made easier.

—John Oliver Hobbes

Nicotine made me numb. With all my stuffed and stuck feelings, I lived mostly in my head. My internal conversation was not easy or constructive. My mind was often too busy with lies and excuses to have an honest and responsible dialogue with myself. Like my outward smokescreen barrier, smoking created a mental fog, a confusion that kept me from seeing the truth.

I took an important action in my recovery when I began working with a sponsor who has put in the time and the commitment to work his recovery program. He offers me experience, strength, and hope on a one-to-one basis. This is also working my Fifth Step.

Some of us need a sponsor to cut through our BS. Some of us need an encouraging word. Some sponsors guide us through uncharted waters and make our way easier by pointing out the rocks and sand bars where we could run aground. And some put the wind in our sails when we are out of breath.

Today, I talk to my sponsor to find support and clarity.

Making amends also means forgiving myself.
—Nicotine Anonymous Member

I felt shame and guilt for what I had done to my son. I had already made amends to him, but not to myself. As I was working on Step Five, my sponsor helped me see that I hadn't forgiven myself. I admitted this shortcoming to my Higher Power. With sincere prayers, I came to honestly forgive myself.

My son and I hadn't talked for several years, yet when the announcement appeared that he was going to be a father, I left him a message with great joy in my heart. He replied, "Thanks," and I was totally amazed.

With great courage and faith, I responded back and we enjoyed a long talk. In my heart I know that this reunion was happening because I have been working the program. I admitted my powerlessness, came to believe in my own Higher Power and worked on doing HP's will for me. I have seen my part in past troubled relationships and have forgiven myself. For the first time in my life, I feel good about myself and the spiritual path I'm on.

Today, I let go, let God, and reap the miracles of recovery.

MAY 4

So many people in my past only knew me as a smoker,
and without recovery. They "missed" me.
—Nicotine Anonymous Member

Recently I was sorting through a box of my memorabilia. There were some objects and photos that got me thinking about the people I knew when I was smoking. Some were from high school, others college, and others from different jobs I had.

The more I thought about it, I realized there were many people in my past who never knew me as a person in recovery. My father died before I got into recovery. People only knew the person behind a smokescreen. I wonder how all those relationships might have been different. We didn't really know each other, not as well as we could have.

Today my relationships are more authentic, more intimate, less anxious, and less judgmental. I still have moments when my shortcomings emerge. These moments are opportunities for growth and healing. I see myself for who I am. I let others see and know me for who I have come to be. I am a grateful recovering nicotine addict, practicing the principles of Nicotine Anonymous, and working toward my own spiritual awakening.

Today, I am grateful I have a presence
and am present with others.

MAY 5

It is easy to stand a pain, but difficult to stand an itch;
it is easy to stand the bitter taste,
but difficult to bear the sour taste.
—Chang Ch'ao

During the last years of my addiction, I had been continuously aware of the pains in my chest, the shortness of breath, and the hacking coughs. I thought I could stand the pain. But I couldn't seem to deal with the urgency of the craving—the nagging, gnawing itch to use nicotine. Over the years, the taste of tobacco became more bitter. It didn't taste good at all. Regardless, I continued to inhale the toxins. Yet, I couldn't bear the sour tasting thought of depriving myself of something I was so dependent on to get through my day.

Now, while working my Fifth Step and admitting the exact nature of my wrongs, I get a clearer perspective on what is healthy and the next right thing for me. When my choices are focused on my recovery and my serenity, I feel more at ease and life is sweeter.

Working the Twelve Steps with my sponsor, doing service work, reading the literature, reaching out to others, and attending meetings are all ways I can focus on my recovery. My new priority of self-care is healing my body, mind, and spirit. The sweetness of life is returning.

Today, I have a clearer perspective
of what is healthy and right for me.

MAY 6

Our inventory also included our good qualities, our assets,
which, when we first stopped using nicotine,
may have been almost impossible for us to see.
—Nicotine Anonymous: The Book

Recovery is a process, which began when I ended my nicotine use. It was like using an ice pick to chip away at my addiction. I still continue chipping away at my character defects. Little by little the process becomes more rewarding as the sculpture of my true self is created and revealed. I work at it in meetings by admitting my shortcomings. I answer the questions in The Questionnaire section of *Nicotine Anonymous: The Book* as well as in the *Nicotine Anonymous Step Study Workbook*. I discuss my responses with my sponsor. More is revealed as I do service work, apply the Traditions to my relationships, and reach out to newcomers.

I may have started with an ice pick but now it's more like shaving the ice—using the many Tools of the program to shape and restore me into the person I want to be.

Today, I am a living art form, at which I continually work.

MAY 7

We discovered that our troubles and tribulations
were just part of the human condition.
We were not awful. We were humbled to realize
that we were normal—and just very human.

—Nicotine Anonymous: The Book

I laughed when I first heard a member share that fellowship meetings are like coming to a surprise party. Then I smiled as I thought how deeply true that was. One of the essential values of attending meetings is experiencing an unexpected truth revealed in the words of a fellow member, or even in my own words. Meetings are safe places to receive these surprise gifts.

Over the years of showing up at meetings, I have learned and confirmed a lot about myself and being human. Being in acceptance of my errant human ways has become a common practice, and hearing others' willingness to admit their own humanity continues to be a powerful experience.

There are times when I'm less than psyched to suit up and show up at a meeting. Then I remind myself of the potential surprises that could be revealed. Surprises could come as words of wisdom or an unexpected newcomer who energizes the whole group to focus on our primary purpose. Being very human, we celebrate our recovery together.

Today, I accept life on its own terms
and the surprise party it can be.

MAY 8

Simplicity is the glory of expression.

—Walt Whitman

Sharing at a meeting is a simple way of expressing my feelings. I talk about what is in my heart to relieve me of the pressure of bearing alone what is going on within me.

I share my experience, strength, and hope. My fellow members benefit as much as I do when I discuss my recovery. At times, I don't want to share—times when I really need to step up and discuss what is preventing me from sharing. That *I am as sick as my secrets* is true for this nicotine addict. No more denial.

I also express myself through writing and making phone calls to my sponsor and others in the Nicotine Anonymous fellowship. This practice helps me during a craving or mental obsession. I practice even when I don't need help, so it makes reaching out easier when I am in trouble or tempted to lose my quit.

In this program of honesty, open-mindedness, and willingness, I express my feelings in healthy new ways which support my recovery and my growth on this spiritual path.

Today, I express myself by discussing my issues and feelings.
I reach out because my fellows may benefit as much as I do.

MAY 9

I love my anniversary coins!
—Nicotine Anonymous Member

When I joined NicA, still smoking, I watched as others happily got their anniversary coins. I applauded, but hid other feelings. I felt envy, frustration, anger, or even shame. I wished I didn't care whether or not I would ever get one.

Finally, I admitted those feelings at a meeting. I said that I really hoped to get an anniversary coin someday. That was a breakthrough moment. In hindsight, I realize that admitting the truth became an important part of my process to quit nicotine a few weeks later.

Soon after I got my second-year coin, I celebrated and went on a two-week Caribbean vacation. There were no smoke free laws there. As I ate, I saw people smoking. Memories flashed in my head. I had a momentary thought, "I'm on vacation, who would know. It could be nice to have just one." Then, I remembered what we say at meetings, "One leads to a ton."

When I reached in my pocket to pay the check, I felt my anniversary coin. I held my coin, and felt that my group and Higher Power were with me. I took a walk along the beach, smiling in gratitude for the coin I can keep in my pocket.

Today, my anniversary coin continues to be a most valued and cherished keepsake, for my sake.

MAY 10

If we are deprived of our just due,
we naturally experience emotions of anger.
—Dr. Smiley Blanton

When I was a smoker, I felt like I was entitled to have whatever I wanted. I thought it was justified. In my Fourth Step inventory I took a thorough look at what was going on emotionally in my life when I first picked up nicotine. I remembered my anger and frustration. I shared my writings with my sponsor. Our talk helped me realize how my anger caused me to remain stuck with a general feeling of being due some justice. I accepted those were old issues that had not yet been resolved.

Now, I ask to be healed from old angers that may remain hidden from me, but which still gnaw at my craw. As I begin to live my life without nicotine, I sometimes have flares of anger out of proportion to a situation. I also find there are times I am legitimately angry about something. This is why my prayers and meditations are so important. I need to ask for the wisdom to know the difference between what was and what is.

With great care, I seek to heal old injustices, and the wisdom to recognize reasonable reactions to interactions. Since smoking has clouded my feelings for so long, I continue to accept the help of a sponsor whose experience has already cleared a path before me.

Today, my recovery gives me more clarity
about my angry feelings and the skills
to have more appropriate responses.

MAY 11

The more we are honest with ourselves,
the more inner trust we develop.
—"How Nicotine Anonymous Works"

I now see that my nicotine use was my way of hiding behind a literal smokescreen. Growing up, often my world did not feel safe. I was one of nine children, so physical and emotional boundaries were broken all the time. I could hardly stand up for myself with so many voices to be heard, and I learned to not trust my own inner voice.

At NicA meetings, I finally have a place that lets me finish my sentences. Meetings have become a safe place, a healing space, and a new home. Finally, I am able to let myself out from behind my protective barriers and be heard. I am given time to complete my own thoughts. Without crosstalk or interruption, I feel safe. Listening to others' honesty teaches me by example. I trust others who clearly care about me.

These are gifts that enable me to open up and live in the present without nicotine. Now, I can speak my mind—the good, the bad, and the ugly—without fear. I can trust myself to speak with patience, tolerance, kindliness, and love.

Today, I share my thoughts with trust in myself and others.

MAY 12

Even as your body betrays you, your mind denies it.
—Sara Gruen

I took my health for granted, and lived in a secret denial of guilt and dread that I was wrecking it. The denial took hold even as a child, after my grandfather, a doctor, died of lung cancer from smoking. Nicodemon convinced me I was immune. One of the lies I told myself was that because so many generations on both sides of my family had smoked, my body had adapted. I didn't have any horrible symptoms, so this must be true. The grand hoax strikes again!

Now that I'm in recovery from this insidious addiction, I treasure every part of my body, bless it, and care for it tenderly. This means drinking lots of water, getting my heart rate up aerobically, stretching, eating fresh healthy foods, pausing to breathe, enjoying the moment, resting well, and having some fun.

Honesty, Openness, and Willingness are HOW I broke through the denial that wanted to keep me in the cycle of addiction. I don't take this quit for granted, I celebrate it daily.

Today, I just want to feel good, be happy, and enjoy this amazing miracle of a whole new life in this sweet body!

MAY 13

The chains that break you, are the chains that make you.
And the chains that make you, are the chains you break.
—Anthony Liccione

Because nicotine is addictive, and I'm a nicotine addict, I'm powerless over nicotine. After decades of ingesting the poisons in cigarettes, I admitted I was chained to my addiction. Yet, the cycle of addiction kept me there.

Thanks to this program of recovery, I have found a way to break free of the chains and let go of the nicotine for good. For me, it takes attending meetings, reading literature, doing service work, getting a sponsor, and working the Steps. It takes reaching out to others who understand, allowing them to help me, and helping those in need. This quit takes vigilance, because the addiction is ever waiting for me to provide a sliver of an opening to get me back into the throes of my addiction. **I'm a Puff Away from a Pack a Day**.

This program of recovery and the amazing people in my Nicotine Anonymous group have helped me to break the chains of this insidious addiction, to speak my truth, and to find a whole new way of life. One day at a time. Sometimes one moment at a time.

Today, honesty frees me from the past,
and I can go forward making clear choices.

MAY 14

I used to be two characters, now I am one person
and accept that I'm human.
—Nicotine Anonymous Member

At a meeting one sentence stood out, "It was about getting real and becoming very human." We admitted how many of us had been two characters. The one we presented to the outside world and the other who we were in our inner world. They were not the same and neither one was really who we were. There was the performer, along with the critic about ourselves and others. Too often the world was a stage upon which we acted.

It is helpful to hear others honestly coming to terms with this aspect of our disease of addiction. I want to recover my true self, to become a whole person and accept my humanity. I want to be more comfortable with who I am on the inside and have the courage to be the same person with others.

I no longer want to hide due to fears of inadequacy. I want to accept myself as I am and be among those who accept themselves, with all of us seeking progress not perfection.

---

*Today, I will be one person, indivisible,
with freedom from nicotine, and compassion for all.*

People are just people,
and all people have faults and shortcomings,
but all of us are born with a basic goodness.
—Anne Frank

Step Five says "the exact nature of our wrongs," Step Six, "defects of character," and Step Seven, "shortcomings." Bill W. said these terms all mean the same thing, and he wrote it like this, because he did not like repeating the same words. If that was the case, then why work three separate Steps when the outcome is the same?

So, I came up with my own interpretation. They all mean the same thing, yet each Step approaches my problem areas from a different angle. Step Five, I tell somebody. Step Six, I become willing. Step Seven, I ask my Higher Power for help.

Each Step is an action Step, but our wrongs, character defects, and shortcomings all mean the same thing, yet with various solutions. I have to tell somebody about them, become willing to have my Higher Power remove them, and then ask my HP to remove them.

Through this process, my own inherent goodness is revealed. The behaviors that no longer serve who I am today are removed, and I am free to become the person I have always wanted to be.

Today, as my character defects are removed,
I am freed of the bondage of self, and accept my goodness.

MAY 16

If I am uncomfortable at this moment, do not be concerned.
In a little while it will be okay.
—A Year of Miracles

The last few times that I quit using nicotine, I was sure I would stay stopped. I had all the will and determination to stay stopped, or so I thought. Then the relapses came, one after another. I would get three days, then a week, but I kept picking up. People in the fellowship said **Keep Showing Up**, it would get better.

Then I would relapse again. Members of the fellowship said, "Don't run away." I had to ask myself if I was running away when I used nicotine, because I couldn't see it. One of the reasons I smoked was to escape my problems. Clearly, trying to escape the discomfort of life was not worth the ill health later on.

After honest reflection, I admitted that running away was exactly what I was doing. As I bounced in and out of recovery during my final attempts at a solid quit, I saw the reality of my discomfort was the withdrawal from the highly addictive substance, nicotine.

I used the "Serenity Prayer for Nicotine Users" to face the discomfort and make new choices about how I responded to cravings. Running away from cravings, feelings, and life never worked. Applying the principles of the program, working the Steps, doing service work, reaching out to other addicts, and attending meetings are how I face life on life's terms now.

Today I stay connected to the fellowship
and participate in my own recovery.

MAY 17

I need my audience, my witnesses.
—Nicotine Anonymous Member

A big reason I **Keep Showing Up** at NicA meetings is that I need witnesses. Others may have different reasons, but I value sharing what I am going through in a safe place with people I have come to trust.

Often, my childhood home was not a safe or trusting environment. High school was a similar nightmare. I needed to conceal most of who I was. Transitioning into my adult years, I carried my painful baggage with me. Relief became my compulsive need, but by using the unhealthiest people, places, and things. Among those wrong things that seemed right was nicotine. My life was often chaotic and unmanageable, especially emotionally.

In addition to nicotine and other substances, I've also sought relief by procrastinating, lying, manipulating, exaggerating, and isolating, to name but a few of my misguided survival techniques. Therefore, I need witnesses to testify to and hold me accountable for my attitude and behavior.

So, I come to testify, though not to be judged. Now, it's a relief to put my cards on the table without any up my sleeve. What a relief to be accepted as I am at my NicA meetings.

Today, as my Higher Power is my ultimate witness,
I deal honestly with myself and others.

MAY 18

I realized that my perfectionism was
just another manifestation of never enough.
—Nicotine Anonymous Member

When I wrote my searching and fearless moral inventory, I wanted to show my sponsor a perfect list of my character defects. No matter how thorough, I worried my efforts would not be good enough, and my sponsor would be disappointed I hadn't fessed up to all my flaws.

I anticipated doing Step Five with a mix of hope and trepidation. Would I receive praise or punishment? I admitted to that before we started going through my list. My sponsor said, "You only need progress, not perfection." We then discussed the curse of perfectionism. I admitted I typically couldn't let myself feel satisfied beyond a brief moment. Delving deeper, I realized that staying satisfied didn't feel safe; I would be vulnerable. I feared the proverbial other shoe would not only drop, but kick me first.

I've longed for a lasting sense of satisfaction. Using nicotine was my ineffective attempt. It only provided a short and false sense of satisfaction. Nicotine is a poison delivered with an underlying cloak of shame for the insanity of it all. My sponsor suggested I could list my assets and see how I could build on my successes rather than on what no longer serves me. NicA is not about hurting, it's about healing.

Today, I ***Keep Showing Up*** *for myself*
and I receive the humble satisfaction
of seeking progress, not perfection.

MAY 19

There's nothing either good or bad but thinking makes it so.
—William Shakespeare

In active addiction, I was always obsessed with nicotine. My every waking thought was consumed by using nicotine, or how to get nicotine. I often thought, "All I can think about is smoking. I'll never stop missing cigarettes."

I have learned that the life I want begins with my thoughts. If I work to avoid an addictive, negative, self-defeating mindset, I discover that I can retrain my thoughts.

My mind believes what I tell it, so I pay attention to what I'm thinking. When a self-defeating thought pops up, I replace it immediately with one that is positive and affirms the mindset I would rather have. I replace words like I can't with statements like I can and I am. I talk to myself with love, compassion, and self-care. I use affirmations and prayer to change my thinking. I say the Serenity Prayer over and over. If I admit my negative thoughts to God and ask to have them removed, then I can stop the war in my head and return to focusing on the breath.

Today, I want to change my life,
so I take action to change my thoughts.

MAY 20

This smokescreen I've been wrapped in keeps out
unpleasant facts about how I chose deprivation over plenty,
cigarettes over love, and over anything else.
—Nicotine Anonymous Member

Even though our stories have different details, most have similar emotional bruises behind them. At first, nicotine seemed to medicate them away. It seemed so easy, when I wanted comfort, I had my pet. Here was compliance at my command.

However, over time I found that nicotine did not heal these injuries or provide me with the satisfaction I had sought. In fact, nicotine became a monster I bowed down to every day. I began to realize that nicotine was depriving me of the very things I wanted. Nicotine is a cunning and cruel tyrant. It dresses up in regal style, promises so much, but then tries to rob me of everything. I realize now that I am not in command, it is nicotine that does the demanding.

What I wanted were the feelings of comfort, assurance, and wellbeing. Once the nicotine was out of my system, I was able to feel again. To get clean it took attending meetings, reading the literature, working the Steps with a sponsor, doing service work, developing a conversation with my Higher Power, and maintaining a place of inner peace where I am safe and present.

Today, I use the Tools of my recovery program to satisfy more of what I truly want in my life.

MAY 21

Becoming honest was a way to get free to be who we were.

—Nicotine Anonymous: The Book

When I first quit smoking, my sponsor told me that I was giving myself an incredible gift. I was confused, because mostly I felt pain and fear. She said that I had to take good care of myself and treat myself well.

During my years of struggling to quit, I was very mean and disrespectful to myself. Smoking was my only "treat," and it was a treat I was ashamed of every day, that robbed me of my money and health, and took me away from those who love me.

When I began my quit with Nicotine Anonymous, I practiced being gentler and kinder with myself, taking it easy, and keeping my life and relationships really simple. As the smokescreen lifted, I could honestly see myself as the good person that I am.

When I found myself worthy of my own love, I felt worthier in general, and that my voice mattered. I don't need to hide or justify my existence. I am enough, I am lovable, I take good care of myself, and treat myself well. As the pain and fear dissipate, I let others into my heart.

Today, I listen to myself and admit my truth.
I don't hide behind a smokescreen anymore.

MAY 22

Expose yourself to your deepest fear;
after that, fear has no power,
and the fear of freedom shrinks and vanishes.
You are free.
—Jim Morrison

When I started in the fellowship I had no idea about gifts of recovery, let alone the freedom it would bring. As a former chronic relapser, I was certainly destined to fail if I tried on my own again. I knew and lived that time after time.

With each method I tried, I figured I would get what I needed to stop and then move on with my life. Freedom eluded me when I could not keep a quit.

Then I surrendered and admitted to my Higher Power I needed help to stop. I listened and let the fellowship teach me how to be a successful quitter and stay quit. I admitted my fear of failure, my fear of being imprisoned by nicotine for the rest of my life.

I learned to pray to quit when I was smoking, to be of service when I can, and observe those who choose NOT to use nicotine. Listening to experienced members and practicing what I'm learning has been key to reaching this new freedom. I want to admit and make right what I have done wrong before. I offer service to my group and support to newcomers. Honesty and acts of courage keep me on my path to stay free of nicotine.

Today, I admit how and why I have relapsed before so I can enjoy the rewards of living free of nicotine.

MAY 23

Clarity is power. The more clear you are about what you want
the more likely you are to achieve it.
—Billy Cox

I see myself and others more clearly now that I'm not hiding the truth from myself, others, and my Higher Power. I discover I am capable. I have more self-esteem and confidence in my abilities.

When I think about the years I spent looking at myself and others through the haze of my addiction, I am both sad and grateful. I'm sad because of all of the false beliefs I used to justify my nicotine use. Now I see that these lies poisoned my self-esteem and my relationships.

I'm grateful because I have more clarity and a new commitment to truth. Although life is far from perfect, my relationships are much healthier, and I have a much more positive view of myself. This is what I really want.

Today, I focus on what is true
and avoid the false beliefs that enable my addiction.

MAY 24

If I'm not phoning members,
I'm still trying to stop using nicotine on my own.
—Nicotine Anonymous Member

When I first began attending meetings, no one had a cell phone and some didn't even have an answering machine. Computers? Email? Not yet. Members' ability to connect between meetings was rather limited.

With the increased use of cell phones and email, we gained the ability to connect and exchange support from almost anywhere. Despite the fact that people usually carry their phones with them all the time, still some members struggle with picking up the "500-pound" phone to call another member or sponsor, especially when they are struggling and could use support rather than use nicotine.

As a sponsor, I am pleased when a sponsee or member calls or texts me. It affirms my faith in our Tools and our saying, "It works if you work it." Calls provide me with an opportunity to serve and give back what is given. Conscious contact with other members supports my recovery and continues to keep me connected. I believe that isolation is the illness and connection is the cure.

Today, I listen to fellow members admit their struggles and share their hopes, as I do the same.

MAY 25

You can please some of the people all of the time,
you can please all of the people some of the time,
but you can't please all of the people all of the time.
—John Lydgate

I started smoking because I wanted to fit in. When another teenager asked me if I enjoyed smoking, I said, "Yes!" even though the truth was "No." Throughout my teenage years and into adulthood, I made choices of how to behave to gain the approval of others. Smoking was one of those ways I lied to myself. I had many acquaintances but few friends. I was barely even a friend to myself.

Today as an adult, I sometimes say, "Yes!" when I mean "No." I take on too many commitments, and I try to save the world. I may not be smoking, but I still end up feeling bad about myself. I admit to my sponsor that I struggle with honesty when it comes to telling people no. Why do I seek the approval of others, when all I need is to approve of myself?

Honesty is something that must be practiced. If I practice honesty in all of my affairs, the reward is a sense of wellbeing and my improved self-esteem. The people that matter most in my life are grateful that I am honest with them, even when being honest is not convenient for me or them. Some people may not like it when I say "No." They may not approve, but the important thing today is that I approve of myself.

Today, I communicate honestly with others about how I feel.
My opinion of myself is what matters,
and I feel good about myself.

Inevitably, someone says the words
I've been trying to find for myself.
—Nicotine Anonymous Member

Left to my own ability to find the words to express my truth, I fumbled in my own darkness. I couldn't see past the obstacles of denial and rationalizations. My addiction created a mental habit of avoiding the truth. The truth disrupted my comfort zone, so I just zoned out. It took a lot of mental gymnastics to ignore the fact that using the addictive toxin nicotine, day after day, year after year, was death defyingly insane.

At NicA meetings, we are guided to listen and not interrupt, criticize, or offer unsolicited advice when another member shares. Whether it's a member who has been freed or one still in the grip of nicotine, I often hear them say something that enlightens my mind. In my silent listening, I have an aha! moment. That's when some truth that has been mangled up inside of me is rearranged and suddenly, I get it and share it. It may come as a relief or like a smack upside my head. These moments are all priceless!

On my own, I had never been willing to seek them out. Now, I listen for the wisdom words of fellow members in the comfort of a meeting and I find my truth.

*Today, my ears are open to hear the truthful words
that keep me honest, open, and willing.*

MAY 27

Our deepest fear is not that we are inadequate.
Our deepest fear is that we are powerful beyond measure.
It is our light, not our darkness, that most frightens us.
—Marianne Williamson

I found freedom from nicotine, but stopped attending meetings after my one-year anniversary. Three years later, after my dad died from lung cancer, I started using nicotine again. For eight years, every time I bought more nicotine, it was going to be my last. I lit candles in churches, chewed the gum, tried acupuncture, got hypnotized, offered tobacco during a prayer ritual, but nothing worked. I remained imprisoned by the addiction.

My mom was dying of cancer, so my return to Nicotine Anonymous was an amends to my parents and to myself. I wanted to grieve without anesthetizing my feelings with nicotine.

This time I admitted how I went wrong and I didn't stop going to meetings after my anniversary. I spent this one-year anniversary at my mom's funeral. A member gave me his one-year anniversary coin that day, but I promised to give it back when I returned to the meeting and receive my own. Through grace, I continue to go to NicA meetings and remain nicotine free.

Believing that service is an expression of gratitude, I worked with another member to start a second NicA meeting in our area. I share what I have learned and when I went wrong. Now I make good choices to light my own spiritual path, and light the way for others.

Today, I stay with what works, because wise action creates hope.

MAY 28

The more we are honest with ourselves,
the more inner trust we develop.
Openness calls upon the courage that facilitates change.
Willingness moves us to act. Action generates hope.
—"How Nicotine Anonymous Works"

A member explained I was free to use the group phone list. I figured I was also free not to use it. So, I didn't. I made attempts to stop vaping, even for a few hours, but I couldn't think straight or sort out what I felt. If I called, wouldn't I just feel more uncomfortable? How could I call someone when I didn't know what to say? My inability to converse was unmanageable.

Then, in a meeting we read the pamphlet, "How Nicotine Anonymous Works." It explained that HOW stands for Honesty, Openness, and Willingness. I had been waiting for hope to somehow arrive before I acted. I had it backwards. I've got to call even when I don't know what to say.

I came to realize that the behavior of not calling was similar to hiding behind a vapor screen. Continuing those behaviors, I would remain stuck in my shame. To gain freedom from nicotine, I need to be willing to go to any length for that freedom. Now, when I am unable to sort out what I feel, I accept that it's time to call and admit it.

Today, I keep in touch with my fellow members,
especially when I'm out of touch with how I feel.

MAY 29

I experienced both grief and excitement
when I first let go of nicotine.
—Nicotine Anonymous Member

I suffered even more grief over a longer period of time just anticipating living without nicotine. I've heard there are progressive stages of grief such as denial, anger, bargaining, depression, and acceptance. I can recall experiencing all those to varying degrees.

But then, I wasn't a member of Nicotine Anonymous. I didn't have compassionate care and support of a sponsor to ease my fears of going through the withdrawal period. My moments of excitement then were short lived because I was alone with my belief that quitting, for me, was impossible.

My experience with excitement was quite different after I joined NicA. At meetings, I was inspired by members who had gained freedom, and those who were still in the grip as I was, yet kept showing up with their desire to be free.

Now, my excitement is based on solid Steps and honest sharing with my sponsor. My stages of excitement have progressed from wishful moments, to suspecting the possibility of hope, to believing I could be helped by something good and wonderful, and then to knowing I could have a spiritual awakening as the result. Believe me, the grief fades, and the excitement remains.

Today, gratefully the grief has been lifted.
I realize I haven't given up anything at all.

MAY 30

In our attempt to deal with our feelings of inadequacy and fear, we came to realize that these were normal human feelings.

—Nicotine Anonymous: The Book

The brain has space for both facts and fears. Both are there to help me survive, but only if there is sanity to create a good balance. When I was using nicotine, I knew the facts about its use being a threat to my life. However, the addiction and my shortcomings overwhelmed me with a fear of living without nicotine. My life lacked any kind of sane balance, and was entirely unmanageable. Denial, rather than faith, was my coping mechanism.

It took months of meetings to get my first nicotine free hours. It has taken years of attending meetings to collect facts from others and to listen within myself to create a better balance. With active practice, I experience positive changes which have become new facts to live by. These facts now occupy more space in my brain than before, while fears have less space to run amok.

Being restored to sanity, to better balance facts with fears, has taken time and practice. The willingness to do so comes from admitting my fears, and seeking the help and inspiration of my fellow NicA members. I did not, and do not, recover alone.

Today, I practice the new facts I've learned, comforted by my new faith.

MAY 31

We can chart our future clearly and wisely
only when we know the path
which has led to the present.
—Adlai Stevenson II

My past is a palette of experiences that paints my present. I have a wide range of feelings about events in my past that shaped and were shaped by my behavior and attitudes. Some are events I would be proud to display. Others were shaded by shame, which I typically kept hidden—shrouded in the smog of nicotine. These events had no purpose but pain and disgrace.

Working through the Steps has revealed that all of my past events can have a positive purpose in my life today. My first lesson has been acceptance that I cannot change the past. Second, I extract value from the past by admitting and learning from my mistakes and accomplishments. Third, I make amends for wrongs. Fourth, I deepen my compassion for others who err in their own ways.

I discovered I am not awful. Clearly, I am just very human. I am an array of colors, bright and muted, that I draw upon to make a beautiful new me. I use the lessons learned to make choices on how to paint the picture of my present, a creative practice in the art of living.

---

*Today, I use the Steps and program principles
to create and maintain my spiritual awakening.*

JUNE 1

Were entirely ready to have God remove
all these defects of character.
—Step Six

I did my Fourth Step inventory. I did my Fifth Step with my sponsor, and I thought I was entirely ready for Step Six and to have all my character defects lifted. I soon realized that being entirely ready to have them lifted also meant that I needed to be entirely ready to let them go.

I realized I wasn't willing yet to stop all the behaviors I had listed. I was afraid. I hadn't prepared or practiced at developing positive, moral attributes to replace whatever my defects and dysfunctional defenses had seemed to do for me.

I revisited my inventory and worked with my sponsor to better understand what I needed to learn. I wanted to become entirely ready. I had been impatient to get through the Steps and feel gratified. Instead, I needed to be thorough and feel grateful for each increment of progress. The journey matters. I suggested topics and listened at meetings. Other insights came through prayer and meditation.

I needed to establish a guided pace that would lead me deeper into issues I had typically raced past before. I practiced new ways of interacting with integrity each day. Steadily, I eventually became entirely ready to let go and have my defects lifted.

Today, humbled by this process, I am preparing for the next Step.

JUNE 2

It is our choices, Harry, that show what we truly are,
far more than our abilities."
—J.K. Rowling

The days following putting down the cigarettes, I felt raw all over, like an open wound freshly exposed to air and sunlight. My body worked overtime to begin the healing process. I took in newly available oxygen after all the years of constant irritation from inhaling hot toxins. My metabolism went haywire without nicotine's stimulants. Sleep, appetite, emotions, focus—all were affected as I withdrew from the violence of nicotine.

The addiction gave way, and then I learned a whole new way of being in the world without relying on nicotine as a crutch, an escape, or a friend. New feelings bubbled up at the most inconvenient times. I reacted to the slightest provocation. In one particularly angry moment, my sponsor asked me, "Is this really where you would like to put your energy?" This stopped me in my tracks. You mean I have a choice?

As the healing continued and the veil of smoke lifted, I began to gain clarity about how to be at peace in the moment, and how to choose to be happy, joyous, and free. What I learned is to surrender, to let go, and let the God of my understanding take care of the people, places, and things that are outside of my control, which are just about everything beyond my own nose.

Today, Higher Power, please show me
and help me choose your will for me,
and give me the power to carry that out.

Whenever I've tried to quit before,
it was like putting a finger in the dike,
but then other crazy behavior would
start leaking out here and then there.
—Nicotine Anonymous Newcomer

Addiction is not just about putting a substance in my body. It's also about the behavior of a person who is not at ease with who they are. It's about me trying to use something outside myself to solve an inside problem. I am not a bad person; I've just had my development arrested by nicotine.

The longer I practiced the addiction, the deeper the void grew within. This emptiness increased my neediness. My shortcomings got me in trouble which led me into the temptation to use. I overworked myself into exhaustion, ate until stuffed, or got into a buying spree at the mall trying to fill the God-sized hole. In the long run, short-term solutions caused my problems to return.

If I don't get at the root of the weed, it will grow back and spread. Through the Twelve Steps, I have become willing to learn more about myself, and I ask that all of my craziness change to sane behaviors. In working Step Six, I become entirely ready to have God remove all these defects of character.

Now, in recovery, this hole in my soul can be filled by conscious contact with my spiritual nature. As I make smobriety and serenity my priority, I find it possible to engage life from a place of fullness and contentment rather than neediness and urgency.

Today, becoming more at ease with who I am,
I engage in life from a place of abundance and contentment.

JUNE 4

The best way out is always through.

—Robert Frost

I spent a great deal of time NOT feeling feelings. My fear of what might happen had great power over me. I might explode with anger! I could sink down the rabbit hole of despair and never get out. Having too much joy wouldn't be right with so much suffering around me.

To escape my feelings, I shoved them back down with smoke and disengaged from the reality of what was really going on in my life, that I was killing myself by using nicotine.

When I found Nicotine Anonymous, I heard about doing the next right thing. Here were happy people, joking and laughing, and not smoking at their feelings. Some had tragedy, others elation, plus all kinds of issues happening in their lives; and they were feeling their feelings and not exploding or sinking down rabbit holes. They shared about doing the next right thing as though it was a guide for getting through the cravings, emotionality, and turmoil. I decided to try it.

Now in recovery, often the next right thing is attending a meeting, reading NicA literature, or doing service. I work through the Steps with my sponsor. I begin to trust my feelings, accept them, and then let them go. This is fully living life on life's terms.

Today, I consciously choose to do the next right thing and notice my feelings. I ask my Higher Power for help with accepting my feelings and letting them go.

JUNE 5

I wish I had a magic wand for anyone
who wants to stop the use of nicotine.
The only magic I have is the Tools of the program.
—Nicotine Anonymous Member

When the craving and emotionality are creating "uncomfortability," I attend meetings in person, on the phone, or online. I call my sponsor or someone on my phone list. I reach for Nicotine Anonymous literature, written by fellow addicts, with love and wisdom from the heart. Literature has helped me through many cravings. I find service is a way to practice my powerlessness over this addiction, and put my focus on helping someone else get free.

I am accountable to a Power greater than myself, and it's okay to be human. My responsibility is to use the Tools of the program to support my quit, to live life on life's terms and to find comfort in healthy new ways.

All I have to do is show up and be present, and eventually the magic of the program will *get* me. Recovery from nicotine addiction is a process, accomplished one day at a time.

Today, I use the tools of the program
to live my life happy, joyous, and free.

JUNE 6

When you're finished changing, you're finished.
—Benjamin Franklin

The adage, "If nothing changes, nothing changes" has a powerful meaning. I once found comfort in the consistency of my habits. But one consistency, my addiction to nicotine, desperately needed to be changed because it was killing me.

I could quit smoking, but could not stay quit. To keep my quit, I learned to embrace good changes in my life. That meant moderate exercise, healthy meals, deep breathing, prayer, and meditation among other new ways of living.

My thinking needed to change too. No more negativity, self-pity, dishonesty and selfish motives. To change my thinking, I had to take action to get to gratitude, acceptance, and willingness.

I became entirely ready. I removed smoking paraphernalia and avoided places where I would be triggered to buy nicotine. I organized clutter, so my home was a clean, beautiful place. I changed my spending habits, to alleviate financial stress, and learned to live within my means. Anything that caused me inner stress needed to change, even my thinking. Now, I reach for better-feeling thoughts, one day at a time, one change at a time.

Today, I make positive changes in my life,
I work toward serenity and freedom.

JUNE 7

I like to encourage people to realize
that any action is a good action
if it's proactive and there is positive intent behind it.
—Michael J. Fox

After a bajillion failed attempts at quitting, it finally dawned on me in a Nicotine Anonymous meeting that to successfully put nicotine down, I would have to be ready to plan ahead. That dawning began my journey into recovery by planning for that first day free of nicotine.

I rid my home of any ashtrays, lighters, or anything related to my nicotine habit. I sorted and washed the clothing I would wear the first few days of my quit. In meetings, when I announced the date, I was applauded and told to "Stay in the middle of the herd" and "Take us with you in your pocket." This was reassuring; I had support and the Tools of the program.

I learned about changing routines. I planned that first morning to shower, brush my teeth, dress, have a protein drink, and head out the door. In the car on the way to work, I had mints and gum. I drove a different route. At work, I jumped right in. I planned my breaks and what would happen after work. I drank lots of water.

And I made it through 24 hours! I read "The Serenity Prayer for Nicotine Users" pamphlet many times, asked my Higher Power for help, attended meetings, kept myself busy, prayed, and breathed through the cravings.

Being proactive worked, and the support of my fellow nicotine addicts carried me through the first weeks and months—one day at a time.

Today, I am proactive about going to any length to not light up.

JUNE 8

When the teacher is ready, the student will appear.
—Kenneth J. Bernstein

I love mistakes. As a sponsor, I have learned more from my mistakes than I have from my successes. Being a sponsor is the greatest learning experience of all.

One day I was talking with a sponsee about relapse, and I said that a slip is the first step in a relapse. My sponsee questioned that by asking, "Before a slip happens, isn't there usually a change or a series of changes in an addict's thoughts, feelings, behaviors, and associations? Addicts rarely slip in a vacuum."

Who is the student and who is the teacher? Of course, my sponsee was right. The slip is not the first step, it's the last one. And so, I learned that I was also the student. Now I'm ready to keep expanding my awareness, learning from my mistakes, and growing in recovery.

Today, I notice my thoughts, feelings, behaviors, and associations. I notice what it feels like to move into my Higher Power's will for me.

If you continue to use nicotine even though
you say the Serenity Prayer, then say it again, and again,
and keep saying it while you reflect on
what it means to you, a nicotine addict.
Eventually it will work.

—“The Serenity Prayer for Nicotine Users” pamphlet

Years after my last quit, I found the wisdom of the Serenity Prayer pamphlet still helps me. Certainly, old triggers of fear, anger, and frustration continued to come up in my life. These are normal feelings in life.

Now, I have the wisdom to know the difference in how to respond. I don’t have to turn to nicotine to stuff my feelings or react to triggers. I accept that this too shall pass.

The Serenity Prayer works in many situations. It’s a bridge over troubled waters. I now practice avoiding a knee-jerk reaction to a thought or feeling. The prayer carries me past the yanking chain of triggered reactions into the place of acceptance where I can make a sane choice. The program works when I work it and I remain ready to let it work me.

Today, I say the Serenity Prayer.
And I can say it again and again.

JUNE 10

Your habit of resistant thought is the only thing
that ever keeps you from allowing the things you desire.
—Esther & Jerry Hicks

My resistant thought is a survival technique which keeps me safe, so I don't have to step outside my addiction to nicotine. "I can't quit because..." "I'll quit when..." That's the addiction talking.

Surrender is a means of getting control of my resistant thinking. I learn to trust that all is well, and that using nicotine never solved anything. I become aware of when the addiction is talking, like when it says, "You deserve one," or "Oh, just one puff."

So, I made a pact with myself that I will go to any length to not light up, and to use every resource available to get this quit going, even if I have just 51% willingness to be willing. My life continuously improves, and the things I desire begin to manifest—all I have to do is breathe.

Today, I am aware of the addiction talking in my head.
I pause and choose to accept the craving and ask for it to be lifted.

JUNE 11

One standard tip for checking on yourself
as it relates to self-care
is to pause and practice H.A.L.T.
—Newcomer's Booklet

I abandoned self-care in the throes of my addiction. I spent my energy on feeding my addiction instead of feeding my body, mind, and spirit. It was an endless cycle of coffee and nicotine, late nights, stress, round and round. I was hungry, angry, lonely, and tired all the time. Nutritious food, fresh air, exercise, or an enjoyable lifestyle were not my priority while I scrambled for the next hit of nicotine.

Once I quit, my health greatly improved, as did my attitude and outlook. I began taking better care of myself. I drank lots of water, ate nutritious food, exercised, worked on the Steps, and changed to more positive thinking. I avoided stressful situations and made my quit my number one priority. Medical exams showed improvement over time, which encouraged me to continue to improve the quality of my life.

Taking good care of myself gets easier as I explore what I like and what feels good, now that I can smell the roses. I believe my Higher Power wants me to experience all of life's joys and delights, and feel really good.

Today, I take good care of myself,
so I am ready to fully experience life.

JUNE 12

He who likes cherries soon learns to climb.
—German Proverb

Even when I was using nicotine, I wanted the cherries of freedom from addiction, but I didn't have a ladder to reach them. I tried to imagine the sweetness of those cherries, but I kept putting the bitterness of tobacco in my mouth.

Now, with meetings and recovery, I am learning how to climb to freedom. The Steps are my ladder. I see that to stop using nicotine and, more importantly, to stay stopped, requires a program of recovery. Meetings offer me the chance to listen to the words of my fellow recovering members. With time, I too will plant new seeds for others to reap the sweet fruit of recovery.

I accept that I can't completely prevent cravings for nicotine that could tempt me to use tobacco. I cannot erase my addiction. I am entirely ready to accept that I need to develop new skills and a relationship with a Higher Power so I can climb up that ladder and keep tasting the sweetness that life has to offer.

---

*Today, I apply the Twelve Steps to my life on a daily basis,
and practice the principles of the program
to the best of my ability.*

JUNE 13

Inspiration exists, but it has to find us working.
—Pablo Picasso

When I first began to seriously think about stopping the use of nicotine, I realized I had spent years struggling to reconcile and rationalize my inability to quit. No matter what other successes I accomplished, I was reminded of my failure when typically, 40 times a day, I lit up. I sucked in failure along with the toxins.

By coming to meetings, I am awestruck by how a simple gesture or sentence that someone shares can be the impulse that motivates me to take a baby step. It is through this process that I discover that I am susceptible to inspiration.

If I show up, miracles can happen. As I open to the understanding and support of fellowship, I find that there are inspiring impulses all around me I hadn't seen before. I surrender, stop struggling, and find relief. I work the Steps and find the inspiration to change my attitude and outlook. In service to others, I apply the Traditions, and am motivated to continue the work; the inspiration continues.

Today, I am open to inspiration that lifts me out of darkness to see myself as I really am.

JUNE 14

Most of the fear that spoils our life
comes from attacking difficulties
before we get to them.
—Dr. Frank Crane

Before I even made an attempt to quit, I spent a lot of time in apprehension, worrying about coping without nicotine. This response to potential difficulties has been a well-worn rut in my life. I worried about many things that never occurred the way I feared they would. I put a lot of time and effort into trying to control situations that I could not control.

At times, my anticipation had me feeling I was experiencing the difficulty before it may or may not have happened. I realized worrying also provided me with excuses not to fully engage with life. I kept one foot in and the other out.

Recovery doesn't mean I can prevent feelings of apprehension from arising. This is when I can ask for the serenity to look at the situation clearly and accept the things I cannot change. Then I ask for the courage to change how I respond. From this calm strength I can improve my chances of getting out of my ruts and being restored to sanity.

Today, I courageously respond to life as it is right this moment.

I'm setting a date to quit.
I don't know if I can make it,
but I'm setting a date.
—Nicotine Anonymous Member

Using nicotine keeps me stuck in an endless cycle of discouragement. It seems that no matter what I think or do, I cannot get off the despair-go-round.

When I attend meetings and witness other members' actions of hope, I begin to believe I can set a quit date. I may continue to struggle with doubt and delay, but I've learned that doubt and delay are colluding cousins in this addictive system.

Setting a quit date can be like casting out a rescue line. It's an attempt to hook something solid, so I can pull myself from the quicksand. If the day comes and I don't make it all the way, I **Look for the Lesson** to learn what I need to do differently. Then I coil up the line, set another date, and cast again.

I'm told there are no failures, just attempts. Attempts are valuable practice. The addict voice in my head may chatter with discouragement. It doesn't want me to break free. I can acknowledge that voice, but not obey it. When this addiction is lifted, none of that noise will matter. I am getting ready.

Today, there are no failures, only opportunities to learn.

JUNE 16

Every conviction was a whim at birth.
—Heywood Broun

Somewhere along the road of my addiction I had a lighthearted whim and admitted, "Ya know, someday I'd like to stop chewing tobacco." I continued on my way and reasons for quitting mounted. In time my whim became a nagging refrain, "I've got to quit, I've just got to stop this."

Then I had the continual, "Damn, I wish I could stop." Eventually the whim became a desire to quit. Thankfully this was also a point where I became willing to reach out for help, and I was able to find it.

I searched the internet and found Nicotine Anonymous. The website said anyone who had a desire to quit using nicotine was welcome. As I faithfully showed up at meetings, my desire developed into a willingness to live without nicotine. At first, I wasn't convinced I would be able to do it, even as I abstained for my first few clean days.

The more I became willing to go to any length to stay nicotine free, the more I became convinced that I could do it, one day at a time. The more I use the program to support my desire, the more I will realize my dream to remain free from nicotine.

Today, with willingness and faithful actions,
I have found a process that makes
my hopes become a reality.

JUNE 17

I'd rather attempt to do something great and fail,
than to attempt to do nothing and succeed.
—Robert Schuller

My first attempt to quit using nicotine is one of the most difficult challenges I've known. Breathing through the fear when it is so fresh and accepting the cravings for the first time is a huge accomplishment. If it was easy, I think more people would be saving themselves from nicotine's deadly clutches.

The anticipation of failing to stop and stay stopped has been more than enough to prevent me from even making an attempt. I know most people are not successful the first time they try to quit nicotine or even the first few times. Other Nicotine Anonymous members tell me, "Recovery is a process, not an instant leap.

Going to meetings to connect with my fellow members helps me to keep working at this process. I'm told failures do not mean defeats. I hear members share the truth of how they slipped and smoked. But then they reflected and learned what tripped them up. I am guided now to study any stumbles rather than use them as excuses. I **Look for the Lessons**.

If I attempt nothing because I fear the failure, I will end up carrying that fear in my pocket for the rest of my life. So, I take a leap of faith and whatever happens, I have the caring support of my fellow members. If I stay ready and accept the process, I will make progress—success I can build on.

Today, I find success in each attempt I make
to move forward in my recovery,
no matter the outcome for today.

JUNE 18

The way to bring about change is to be proactive and active.
—Octavia Spencer

I quit at 8 pm on a Sunday night, and immediately attended an online meeting. I had to be proactive about my quit and totally change my routine. My quit became the number one priority.

I had a plan. Getting up in the morning, I jumped in the shower first, and had a protein shake before heading out the door. No lingering over coffee. I had mints and gum stashed in the car, because driving was a trigger. And I drove a different route to work to avoid driving by the tobacco shop.

At work, I had my coffee. I had a stash of chewing gum at my desk, and I drank jugs of water. On break, I walked for 10-15 minutes before returning to my desk. I used earphones to listen to NicA meetings and carried the names, phone numbers, and email addresses of folks in the program. I brought literature to work to read during lunch, and then brushed my teeth and took a brisk walk after eating. The minute I got home from work, I jumped into the discussion board, attended meetings, emailed my sponsor, and checked in with friends in NicA. By 8 pm I had another 24 hours, and celebrated with tea and cookies.

For me, going to any length to not light up required planning, intention, perseverance, and celebration.

Today, I am proactive about my quit,
ready to make my recovery the top priority in my life.

JUNE 19

As a newcomer, each meeting I attended
put another log on the fire of my desire.
—Nicotine Anonymous Member

When I first arrived at a Nicotine Anonymous meeting, I had maybe a 10% desire to stop using nicotine. My other 90% was a mix of doubt that it was possible to stop and a fear of how I could cope without nicotine.

In meeting after meeting, we read from the literature, sometimes about a Step, sometimes a pamphlet. I heard this is a WE program and a slogan, **Together We Change**. I listened as others shared things I could identify with. I began to bond with the group and my desire grew week by week, because of what we read and the sharing I heard.

The other members' efforts and enthusiasm inspired me to hope. My desire to gain freedom from nicotine kept increasing. I truly began to suspect the possibility that I would one day escape my obsessively addicted ways.

I realized that if I had stayed alone without meetings, my desire to quit would never have grown to be ready to let go of nicotine. It is said recovery is a process, not a sudden event. For me, this process included consistently showing up for meetings and adding more logs to the fire of my desire until, yes, I got free.

Today, I celebrate the fire of my desire to live free of nicotine.

JUNE 20

The greatest test of courage on earth
is to bear defeat without losing heart.
—Robert Green Ingersoll

A nicotine relapse feels like a defeat, a failure. Despite my desire to stop using nicotine for 20 years, many mornings started with the feeling of defeat when I relapsed and, yet again lit another cigarette. I was alone with my desire to stop.

When I joined Nicotine Anonymous, I found that I was no longer alone. At first, I did not have the courage to go through withdrawal. Yet, just being present, listening and being accepted by the group members was enough for me to **Keep Showing Up** and not lose heart. Little by little, I borrowed courage from the example of other members.

After several months, I hit bottom when I failed another quit date. But because of the group support, that bottom was less about losing heart and more about a final surrender. Within days, I became willing to delay smoking, this time starting with two hours nicotine-free. I so wanted to make it to the next meeting and give them the good news.

Decades later, the courage I borrowed, and now practice daily, still serves me well in my life's endeavors. I serve NicA and **Keep Showing Up**. Nicotine hasn't defeated me again, and my heart is hopeful.

Today, I live with gratitude for this freedom
and the courage to do what I thought I never could.

JUNE 21

Tyranny is a habit capable of being developed,
and at last becomes a disease.
—Fyodor Dostoyevsky

When I became angry enough at being tyrannized by my own addiction, I finally became ready and willing to quit using nicotine. I had thought I just had a smoking habit, but smoking became a force that owned me and enslaved me. It was the center of my life and had squeezed out my spirit and my breath, as if the nicodemon had sat heavily on my chest.

Living nicotine free is being truly free to connect with my own spirit, with others, and with my Higher Power. I am also free to connect with my core values, my creative spirit, and my desire to grow spiritually. With freedom from the tyranny of nicotine, I have also grown more prosperous in my relationships, my finances, and my ability to be grateful.

Nicotine Anonymous has helped me heal from the terrible effects of addiction, and find true freedom in body, mind, and spirit.

Today, I am truly grateful for my freedom.

JUNE 22

Self-pity in its early stage is as snug as a feather mattress.
Only when it hardens does it become uncomfortable.

—Maya Angelou

"Woe is me" is a classic expression of self-pity. Before I attended Nicotine Anonymous meetings and began practicing program principles, I could slide into self-pity as easily as into a comfortable old shoe. When I was lonely or felt a lack of anything in my day, self-pity was right there, just like my nicotine—always within reach.

Using the *Nicotine Anonymous Step Study Workbook*, I discovered how self-pity was an ineffective character trait. My answers revealed how self-pity was not a solution, but another problem. I realized that whenever I made efforts to stop using nicotine, I kept slipping up because I had slid into self-pity. Just as nicotine seemed to help me feel better temporarily, self-pity seemed to do the same. What I actually lacked in my life was something or somewhere better, healthier, to go to in order to soothe my feelings.

To live happy, joyous, and nicotine-free, and make my life more manageable, I acknowledge self-pity as one of my shortcomings. Admitting this helps me become entirely ready for this character trait to be removed. I pause and seek comfort and inspiration by making conscious contact with a source of grace. I ask this source for the mercy that comforts me and the courage to change the things I can.

Today, I say, "Whoa, I have a better place to go."

JUNE 23

I chose the integrity of withdrawal
rather than the insanity of addiction.
—Nicotine Anonymous Member

For years, just my thoughts about nicotine withdrawal symptoms brought on feelings of panic and despair. I rarely forgot to keep a supply of nicotine on hand. As laws changed and limited where I could smoke, I was forced to experience moments of withdrawal. That was when finding a place where I could smoke became a top priority. Some of those times I was in a state of mania. I lost my self-respect and integrity in the insanity of my addiction. I wanted to stop, but the panic created a powerful urgency.

Deeply demoralized, I turned to NicA as a possible solution. I was a member of another 12-Step fellowship, which had helped restore me to sanity, but clearly not completely. For months, I attended NicA meetings and shared, often tearfully about my stressful life and fears. Yet, as I listened to hope, I felt care and support.

Finally, I took that leap of faith into withdrawal. I wasn't alone. I had my group, literature, and my awakening spirituality. Yes, there were tough times, but I was honest and true to myself. I was strengthened by an integrity that I've learned to value over the insanity of ingesting nicotine's toxins. I am free to become the person I always wanted to be.

Today, I choose the integrity of living without nicotine rather than the insanity of using it.

JUNE 24

Always say 'yes' to the present moment…
Surrender to what is. Say 'yes' to life—
and see how life starts suddenly
to start working for you rather than against you.
—Eckhart Tolle

By myself, I could not quit no matter what scheme, tool, product, or strategy I used. I needed help. Surrendering was how I was able to get my Higher Power's help. I let go, allowed myself to be open to receiving, and God was there. I sincerely asked for help, and the God of my understanding responded, and I found Nicotine Anonymous meetings.

An hour into my quit, I stood in the hallway looking up at the ceiling and pleaded with my Higher Power to help me through a craving. I breathed and I prayed. Nothing happened. The craving passed, and all was well. I thought, "Ha! Take that ol' Nicodemon!" I had a power much greater than the addiction helping me through the craving.

When craving, emotionality, turmoil or unmanageability hit, tips like the 5 Ds—Delay, Distract, Discuss, Drink water, Deep breathe— come in handy. Another tip is to stay in the middle of the herd, reach out and find support. "The Serenity Prayer for Nicotine Users" pamphlet keeps me focused and practicing acceptance of the cravings and changing the way I respond to them. **Smoking is Not an Option**, no matter what.

Today, getting free of nicotine is doable
if I surrender and use tools to build my new nicotine-free life.

JUNE 25

Great things are not done by impulse,
but by a series of small things brought together.
—Vincent Van Gogh

I wanted this compulsion to use nicotine to stop. Just stop! I wished the craving would disappear. I had met people who said that one day they simply decided to stop using nicotine, and that was that. Why was it so difficult for me?

I had questions, without answers. I only saw my inadequacies. That emptiness was filled by fear and negativity. One fateful day, I noticed a flyer about Nicotine Anonymous. Desperate, I showed up. I listened and read. I found people with similar stories, some still seeking freedom or others who had found it. I began to feel the possibility of hope.

After attending meetings for several months, a moment came when I was finally willing to forego the next one until later. Although I previously wished for a sudden impulse, what worked for me was a series of small things, the sequence of the Steps that moved me forward.

I found the answer. I stopped comparing myself to others and started identifying with others who inspired me to be more than I had been and to improve myself. Once I resolved to focus on this program's solution, I had a plan and a process to change and be healed.

Today, I continue to do the little things
that have led me to big improvements.

JUNE 26

Every thought I have imprisoned in expression,
I must free by my deeds.
—Kahil Gibran

So many times I had thoughts about quitting nicotine. I wrote them down in journals or spoke them aloud to friends. At times, this relieved some pressure; I thought I had good intentions. Other times, it only increased my frustration and self-loathing.

Occasionally, I would stop for a while and be let out of my prison for a reprieve. However, left to my own devices, I would eventually return to the scene of my crime. There I would be caving to the craving, caught and convicted, and sentenced to my isolated cell, waiting to be put on death row. I had good intentions, but I did not have a step-by-step plan to achieve freedom.

When I discovered Nicotine Anonymous, I read that the Twelve Steps offered a process of specific actions that I could take and deeds I could do. I saw others get "paroled" and set free from nicotine. Until I discovered this program of recovery, none of my good intentions could free me.

As a nicotine addict, I accept that intentions are idle. I note the actions that have worked for others, and take them to get results and achieve goals.

Today, I follow up good intentions with timely actions.

Feelings or emotions are the universal language
and are to be honored.
They are the authentic expression
of who you are at your deepest place.
—Judith Wright

I never learned how to effectively deal with feelings, and I found they can often be overwhelming. Using nicotine, I stuffed the feelings back down, never dealt with them, and became fearful of my feelings. So, I hid behind the smokescreen, and my dependence on nicotine grew stronger, all the while killing me softly.

In recovery, to get in touch with my feelings, I breathe, get very quiet, and find where the feeling is in my body. When I locate the feeling, I sit with it just for a few minutes, rest with it, accept it. Then I am able to let go of the feeling and move on.

It's pretty simple. Often, when I sit with the feeling, come to rest in it, the feeling dissipates and loses its power over me. Usually, I am very tender with myself as I work through feelings.

I often write out what comes to mind, or draw to visualize it. Many times, after resting with my feelings, I work through my part and make an amends. Often, I use sticky notes with affirmations in places I frequent (mirror, computer screen, or dashboard) to help me change my thinking. Every time I practice this process, I feel better afterwards.

*Today, I accept my feelings and consciously choose
the direction of my thoughts.*

Keep practicing your recovery behaviors,
even when they feel awkward,
even when they haven't quite taken yet,
even if you don't get it yet.
—Nicotine Anonymous Member

I accept it can take years for a recovery concept to move from my mind into my heart and soul. I work at recovery behaviors with diligence, effort, and repeated practice. I do things even when they don't feel natural. I tell myself I care about myself and I practice self-care, even when I don't believe what I'm saying.

I *act as if* for months and years, before recovery behaviors become ingrained and natural. Even after long periods, in times of stress, I may find myself reverting to old ways of thinking, feeling, and behaving.

It takes time and repeated practice to get self-love into the core of my being. Then, just when I think I've arrived, I find there's more to learn. That's the joy of recovery. I get to keep learning and growing all my life!

So, I keep loving and taking care of myself, no matter what. I tell myself to focus on recovery one day at a time, even when it doesn't feel natural. I *act as if,* even if that time period seems long.

One day, it happens. I wake up and find that what I've been struggling with and working so hard at, finally feels comfortable in my soul. Then I go on to learn more on this spiritual path.

Today, I patiently work at my recovery,
trusting I can change the things I can,
and have the peace that I seek.

JUNE 29

It needs courage to throw oneself forward;
but it needs not less to hold oneself back.
—Désiré Joseph Cardinal Mercier

The Serenity Prayer has an order to it just as the Steps do. In order to receive the courage to change the things I can, I first need the serenity to accept the things I cannot change. It is from this place of centered calm that I can see clearly where to focus the courage I receive. I can be more confident that my efforts are worthwhile. Without serenity I will be frustrated, confused, and open to anxiety.

Sometimes I need the courage to move forward in a new way. Other times I need the courage to stop myself from doing what I've done in the past. Now, instead of picking up nicotine or practicing a shortcoming, this courage can put off my old reflex action until it passes.

I cannot change the fact that I crave nicotine. This is how I am and how my body is. In this acceptance, I find peace and wisdom to make choices with courage.

To go forward is an act of faith that moves me away from my shackles of fear. Even when I think saying the Serenity Prayer won't help, I say it. I give peace a chance.

Today, when I begin with serenity,
I have the courage to make wise choices.

JUNE 30

I'm entirely ready to look into my cracks
and see what they reveal.
—Nicotine Anonymous Member

Initially, when it came to actually working the Twelve Steps, my shortcoming of procrastination enabled my inaction. However, the honesty and soul-searching of other members helped me admit to my fear-based behavior. I had justified ignoring the evaluation of my shortcomings as an unpleasant, painful and shameful exercise. I had not wanted to believe a Fourth Step had useful value. As *Nicotine Anonymous: The Book* points out, "we really did not want to look all that in the face."

Once I had a few months nicotine free, I became concerned about how easily one or more of my shortcomings could cause me to relapse. So, I began my inventory. I realized that these defects of character could provide me with insight into how and why I so often ended up where I didn't want to be or feeling what I didn't want to feel.

I used the program's Tools and the *Nicotine Anonymous Step Study Workbook*, and began to make sense of my insanity. With spiritual care and group support, I came to see what I could not see on my own. As the air is clearing, my mind is clearing, and I'm moving forward with mending my life.

Today, I continue to look for cracks that reveal
what I need to look into.

JULY 1

In my Seventh Step, I humbly ask my Higher Power
to remove my shortcomings.
—Nicotine Anonymous Member

The God of my understanding provides me with serenity, courage, and wisdom to heal my body, mind, and spirit from this terrible disease that kills so many. In my Third Step, I made a decision to turn my will and my life over to the care of a God of my own understanding. However, this does not mean that I don't have anything to do. Recovery is a cooperative venture with my Higher Power, the fellowship, and me. I was given the gift of precious life: a body to care for, a mind to learn with, and emotions to feel life's experience.

I'm reminded of a Russian proverb, "Pray to God, but keep rowing to shore." I row because I need exercise to strengthen my body. I row to accept the responsibility for my life. I row to feel connected to my journey and my spiritual path.

As I humbly ask my Higher Power to remove my shortcomings, I become more aware of my strengths. I build on my strengths as I continue with the work. With my Eleventh Step, I ask for knowledge of my Higher Power's will for me and the power to carry that out, guiding me on my way. I row to shore so I can keep focused on my goal of being happy, joyous, and free. I do the work because I am worth it.

Today, I cooperate with my Higher Power,
and I do my part for my recovery.

JULY 2

Smoking Is Not An Option.

—Nicotine Anonymous slogan

Taking Step One, "We admitted we were powerless over nicotine— that our lives had become unmanageable," is where I woke up to the fact that I had no control over my use of nicotine. My whole life focused on getting the next hit. At first, I couldn't see the unmanageability because I thought it was normal behavior for smokers, having been exposed to nicotine from birth onward.

I wanted it when I wanted it, and my life became one powerless drag off the death stick to the next and the next, to the point of feeling so awful physically, emotionally, spiritually that I finally hit bottom.

The worst part of the unmanageability was the dishonesty, shame, and guilt. I am so happy to have asked and had that enormous weight lifted from my heart and shoulders.

I am still powerless over nicotine, and always will be. Happily, a Power greater than myself has helped me, the Tools of the program have empowered me, and my friends in the program have supported me through the rough stuff.

Today, I find comfort and serenity
in my powerlessness over nicotine.

JULY 3

As the numbness lifts, we begin to feel again,
sometimes to the temporary peril of those around us!
—"Our Promises"

When I got my quit going, I went to a lot of meetings; I told my loved ones that for the next little while, I would need to focus on my quit above all else. Life could not go on as it had before. I had to be proactive about the changes, and ask others for patience, tolerance, kindliness, and love as I moved through withdrawal and into my new life.

Recovery had to be totally selfish for me to get this quit going and keep it going. There were times when my anger roiled, or I was in tears over the slightest thing. I was experiencing feelings for the very first time.

There was much discomfort over that, because facing these everyday human feelings was so new; I had ol' nicodemon roaring in my ears badly wanting me back. But my friends in Nicotine Anonymous, especially my sponsor, helped me and carried me through the wild storms of withdrawal and early recovery. I heard that if you're feeling, you're healing.

It really helped to be honest about where I was, and to ask for help and support. It's the hardest thing I've ever done—it was like giving birth to a new me!

Today, I am aware of, and accept my feelings
with gratitude that the numbness was lifted.

JULY 4

Everyone needs help. That's the human condition.
—Max Allan Collins

In my twenties, after a few years of smoking, I had the desire to quit. Yet I was unable to do so because I feared being incapable of dealing with life on life's terms. This likely was my addiction talking. After 30 plus years of smoking a pack a day, I hit bottom terrified and hurting, and I pleaded with my Higher Power for help.

After that foxhole prayer, I realized I had the desire to quit, I just needed courage and support. I reached out and a Power greater than me led me to Nicotine Anonymous, whose members showed me the Steps to freedom. I found an online NicA meeting, where the support of my fellow addicts bolstered my courage to look at the reality of my addiction. I found strength to face the fatal attraction. I stayed in the middle of the herd with those who had gone before me, those who knew how to deal with the addiction to nicotine. I moved through the fear and into freedom from nicotine.

I feel that my ability to go to any length to not light up has been a community effort. It has taken support from my significant other, friends, family, fellow nicotine addicts, colleagues, and even strangers to help me get this quit going and lift this addiction from my life.

During the early days, I began developing a relationship with my Higher Power. And still today, as I deal with life on life's terms, I allow others and my Higher Power to help and care for me. I cannot do this alone.

Today, I have the courage to reach out when I need help, and to listen for my Higher Power's will for me.

JULY 5

God has devised ways for all of us to live,
but it is for us to choose how.
—Neeraj Singhvi

I've got to love myself first. And the next right loving thing I can do for me is to quit using harmful substances like nicotine. Another way is to fill my thoughts with positivity. I'm attracting whatever I think, so when I think happy thoughts, I'm a magnet for the good stuff in life. Thinking positive thoughts is a way to love myself.

Another loving act is to become aware of when I'm entrenching myself in fear or other negative thinking. Once I have the awareness, I can begin to change my thinking. For me, it has taken a kind of brainwashing to replace the negative thoughts with positive ones, over and over until my thinking changes.

A negative thought might be, "Oh no! This person might be mad at me and not like me anymore!" I can replace that fear-based thinking with a positive affirmation: "I am loving and kind and doing the best I can for myself and all concerned."

Affirmations are simply statements that state what I want in the present tense. A power greater than me provides whatever I ask for. Fear or abundance? Feel good or feel bad? It's up to me.

Today, I love myself
and focus on the goodness life offers.

JULY 6

Our soul can be robbed of its power by resentment.

—Pir Vilayat Inayat Khan

Before recovery, I sucked my anger down with drags of nicotine. That anger festered into resentments. My resentments usually operated under cover. Whenever I quashed my feelings, I wasted energy digging tunnels to bury them. That gave me a false sense of managing. Where was the joy in my life?

Recovery has shown me that it's my responsibility to respond to daily events in appropriate ways. One way is to pause, breathe, and allow my Higher Power between me and whatever is provoking an angry response in me.

I now see that anger can have value as a signal that something is wrong. If I have acted out in anger, the task is to address such situations appropriately. I seek collaborative solutions, make any necessary amends when possible, and I don't submerge my anger into resentments.

Working Steps Four through Seven, I identify any festering resentments that I have held onto, share what I learn with my sponsor, then ask that my shortcomings be lifted. I use the Steps to let go of addictive toxic substances and corrosive toxic resentments. And I find a new sprinkle of joy in my life.

Today, I let my healing happen
and embrace life's joys as I recover.

Inaction breeds doubt and fear.
Action breeds confidence and courage.
If you want to conquer fear,
do not sit home and think about it.
Go out and get busy.
—Dale Carnegie

I have spent countless hours in isolation and inaction. I sat, smoked, and drank coffee for most of my day. I let important things pile up and allowed messy clutter in my home. Self-doubt and fear fed the addiction cycle.

Now, with my freedom from nicotine, I have a great deal of time to create changes in my life by taking action. I am actually becoming more confident and courageous now I have quit.

One action I can take is reaching out to help a fellow nicotine addict or asking for help myself. I get out of my own head by reaching out, and I grow spiritually.

Other actions include going to meetings, sharing, reading the literature, contacting my sponsor, and doing service work. I focus on Nicotine Anonymous rather than nicotine. Also, writing helps me find clarity in a situation.

Doubt and fear arise from time to time, so I use these program Tools and take other actions in my recovery. Reciting the Seventh Step Prayer, I ask God to remove the fear or doubt. At any time, I can do a Tenth Step spot check inventory, then let go and let God. Action changes my life for the better!

Today, actions change my thinking,
giving me confidence and courage to stay nicotine-free.

That's it! I'm done! Not one more!
—Nicotine Anonymous Member

Accepting that I am truly letting go of using nicotine is a personal process that I have had to find my way through; it's a journey into the unknown. That is why being in this fellowship is so helpful. My approach has been slow and steady. I've seen how for others the journey has been a wild and bumpy ride. Some have several slips and slides. It took me showing up at meetings for over seven months before I had my first clean day. It takes whatever it takes to say goodbye to nicotine.

From all the people I've witnessed, I'm convinced that whatever the process is, it's exactly the way it needs to be for that person. At times, walking through my fears felt like I was walking the last mile on death row. Actually, I was walking away from the executioner and toward my freedom.

When I reached a point when I became willing to let go and have my chemical crutches lifted, I made a decision not to have even just a few for the day. Soon there was no lingering desire for yet another last kiss of nicotine. I became willing to walk forward and be free. I accepted that the relationship with nicotine was over and said, "I'm done." Now my life is a spiritual journey abundant with appreciation for the recovery process, the people who accept me as I am, and a reverence for my new freedom.

Today, I am surrounded with support and grace,
so I can embrace and cherish my new freedom.

JULY 9

The opposite of addiction is connection.
—Johann Hari

Quantum physics explains that everything in the universe is connected; nothing can exist separately. The universe exists because of this interaction. There is even beauty in what appears to be chaos.

Every atom, molecule, person, place, and thing is subject to, and in a process of, transformation. The wisdom in Nicotine Anonymous supports transformation through connection with our fellows and by seeking to improve our conscious contact with a Higher Power we each understand. Our pamphlet, "Our Policy of Openness," affirms that personal journey of spiritual awakening.

I see marvelous mystery and chaotic mayhem in the universe, in this fellowship, and in my own life. All are connected. Yet, my free will allows me to choose a path that either embraces connection or attempts to avoid it. I choose a spiritual path that embraces this principled desire of connection.

Our Seventh Step Prayer seeks this embrace: "My Higher Power, I place myself in your hands and humbly ask that my character defects be lifted from me so that I may help others. Please grant me willingness, courage, and strength so that through my actions I may reflect your love and wisdom. Amen."

Today, I connect with willingness, courage, and strength;
and, I embrace my Higher Power's will for me.

JULY 10

And so rock bottom became the solid foundation
on which I rebuilt my life.
—J. K. Rowling

Even before I joined Nicotine Anonymous, I had heard that an addict may have to hit rock bottom before recovery begins. I identify with this idea because I struggled to stop using nicotine. I agonized about how low my bottom is. I felt I was still falling, hitting rocks along the way. I ached in body, mind, and spirit. If I was not at rock bottom, it was certainly rocky. My lungs hurt from coughing, my mind was consumed with anxiety and self-loathing, and my spirit was without hope.

My thoughts rocked back and forth between *I need nicotine* and *I need to live and breathe.* I was stuck, wishing for a magical intervention, but not willing to go to any length. I continually gave into the craving rather than completely surrendering to seek help.

Discovering NicA was my start. Meeting by meeting I became willing to change. I began climbing back up from those rocks. I didn't want to return to them, yet I didn't want to forget how painful they were. Members reached out with support and showed the way by example. Step by Step I climbed, until I could see hope's light shining above, and I was spiritually lifted up to recover my life.

Today, I practice the principles built on the solid rock foundation of recovery and fellowship.

JULY 11

Physical improvement has been almost immediate.
Our sense of smell and taste returns;
the world takes on a new dimension of color and clarity.
—"Our Promises"

Physical improvement eluded me at first. It seemed that my cough worsened. I was disappointed that I wasn't able to walk faster. Gradually, with the help of my Higher Power, there has been physical improvement. I am active to improve my stamina. I now make healthier lifestyle choices for improving my health and wellbeing.

My sense of smell and taste did return, but I wasn't happy about some of the odors. I had never admitted that my clothes smelled bad. I once thought I had control over my smoking by only smoking in my car. But really, nicotine and my addiction had control over me. Once my sense of smell returned, I could not deny that my car smelled terrible. However, today I don't have to interrupt my day looking for an opportunity to drive somewhere so I can smoke.

I have a new honesty and clearer outlook on the world. Spiritually, I have a growing connection with my Higher Power. This Power helps me clean up my shortcomings so that I may have a longer life.

---

*Today, I am humbly grateful for my physical improvements
and for the ability to stop and enjoy the roses.*

JULY 12

Sometimes all it takes to let go
is the right person to hold onto.
—Steve Hartman

For too many years I held onto my cigarettes for dear life. I came to believe they were my best friends, the companions that would always be by my side or in my pocket. When I reached for help, I reached for a cigarette.

As health concerns and prices increased, my use of cigarettes became a love-hate relationship. When I became a NicA member, I read up on nicotine and all the toxic chemicals in tobacco smoke. After some research, I came to understand that my "love" was due to how nicotine supposedly raised levels of brain chemicals and created the illusion of pleasure for me, which reinforced the bond of the drug, the addiction.

I finally let go of cigarettes because, like my original group members, I had an experienced sponsor who was the right person to hold on to as I walked through the Steps. "Our Promises" rang true: "We now realize we have been participating in a grand hoax." I had not given up anything at all.

Our slogan, **Watch Your Steps**, reminds me that "as an addict, I must beware of slippery places." So, I continue to support, honor and respect this quit, and I remain ever mindful to hold onto the many resources the fellowship provides.

---

*Today, I will let go of illusions, and hold onto what is real—
the Steps and my sponsor.*

JULY 13

Comfort zones are most often expanded through discomfort.
—Peter McWilliams

Any physical or emotional discomfort was a justification for a cigarette. I believed I could not cope with life's discomforts without nicotine, so my desire to get free of nicotine seemed unattainable.

I saw a flyer for a Nicotine Anonymous meeting, but worried it would be uncomfortable to sit through such a meeting. Finally, I decided to go at least once. After all, the only requirement was to have a desire to stop, and I had that.

Soon I asked a member to be my sponsor. I expressed my concerns about dealing with the discomfort of nicotine withdrawal. She shared how she had accepted her discomfort as temporary and part of the change process. She had asked her Higher Power to expand her comfort zone to accommodate withdrawal. She suggested I read the pamphlet, "The Serenity Prayer for Nicotine Users," as a good guide for accepting the discomfort.

The Serenity Prayer provided a sane perspective. It helped ease my concerns about change and discomfort. I asked for my comfort zone to be expanded because the benefits were worth it.

With my wise sponsor's support, I accepted the temporary discomfort of withdrawal, and changed my life completely. Nicotine is no longer an option for me. Now I choose serenity, courage, and wisdom.

Today, I am grateful for this program that helped relieve the discomfort of my addiction.

JULY 14

I may enjoy feeling I've got it licked,
but beware there's no guarantee it'll stick.
—Nicotine Anonymous Member

When I finally started to put a few weeks together clean from nicotine, it was very exciting. I was surprised that refraining from nicotine turned out to be less difficult than I had imagined. I discovered that I was more powerful than I had once thought. I sensed a new enthusiasm about myself and what might happen in my life. I stopped going to NicA meetings thinking, "Thanks, but I got this."

Two months later, I was with a friend who still smoked. I thought I'd have one with him. The next day I bought a pack to have one once in a while. In no time, I was right back to smoking every day. It took a few months before I mustered the courage to return to the meeting.

This time I paid more attention to the program's suggestions for developing and maintaining humility. It is essential to my recovery that I remember Step One to stay nicotine free, and practice Step Seven to stay humble. Clearly, I am powerless over nicotine. With humility, I become right-sized in relation with my Higher Power.

Today, I watch my Steps because
although it may appear I'm out of the woods,
I can still stray off the path.

JULY 15

We begin to forget we had been nicotine users,
except at meetings.
—"Our Promises"

I came to meetings for a while, and it helped me to quit using nicotine. Yet, I stopped going to meetings once I got what I wanted. I thought I didn't really need the program anymore. I thought I had passed the course. After eight years of enjoying life without smoking, I forgot I was a nicotine addict. I went on a weekend camping trip with some friends. The first night around the campfire, one friend was smoking. I said, "Heck, I'm taking time off this weekend; let me have one of those." I thought, "I got this smoking thing under control." I fired one up.

Within a week I bought a carton. I'd gone down the hole again. I remained gone from the meeting for two more years. Finally, humbled, I showed up and thankfully the same members were still there. I was welcomed without judgment.

It took several months, but by the grace of God and the support of my fellow members, I got free again. "Our Promises" made it clear to me what I had forgotten, that I was a nicotine addict, and I had stopped coming to meetings. Now I'm attending meetings, working the Steps and offering service to the group that saved me once again.

---

*Today, I reaffirm my commitment to **Keep Showing Up**,*
lest I forget what I need to remember about my addiction.

JULY 16

A man's worst difficulties begin
when he is able to do what he likes.
—Thomas Henry Huxley

As a kid I was frustrated that I couldn't do all I wanted. So, I figured out clandestine ways and took risks for excitement. I started using tobacco when I was underage, trying to show off to friends how I could do whatever I liked. I used nicotine as my rite of passage, as an act of defiance and protest.

Adults said not to use nicotine even while they did. It looked like they got to do whatever they liked. The rules didn't seem fair, so I ignored rules, thinking that I had the freedom to get whatever I liked. I made decisions disregarding whether or not they made sense or were safe.

Whatever I may have gotten out of using, it did not satisfy my soul. I became desperate to gain freedom from this disabling prison, and I joined Nicotine Anonymous. I was asked to do service, and though I wanted to ignore responsibility, my soul said yes.

Over time, my addiction was lifted. I developed new abilities and gained a deeper satisfaction than I had ever known. Letting myself be guided by a higher purpose has become a journey of humility and gratitude, qualities I truly want.

Today, I will work Step Seven and humbly ask
that my defiance be lifted.

JULY 17

Don't be concerned with being disloyal
to your pain by being joyous.
—Pir Vilayat Inayat Khan

In my youth, I made numerous errors and suffered painful consequences. I used nicotine to numb my painful feelings. At times, I avoided experiencing joy for fear that it might turn into disappointment and pain. I grew attached to my pain as a familiar partner in life.

Whenever painful or angry feelings arose, I continued to use nicotine to stuff them back down. Resentments bred deep down within me. Resentments made it difficult to let my guard down so I could enjoy feeling good.

My attempts to cope had created character defenses that ultimately kept me insulated from feeling deep joy and love. Our Third Step Prayer opened my heart to "Keep me alert with courage to face life and not withdraw from it, not to insulate myself from all pain whereby I insulate myself from love as well." I began to gain the courage to change the things I can.

In the Sixth and Seventh Steps, I seek the readiness and willingness to have my defects of character lifted, forgive myself, and let go of the pain. As I participate in our fellowship, I embrace joy without fear by practicing the principles of our program.

Today, I let go of my character defects and I am joyous.

JULY 18

Nicotine is an insidious addiction,
and in NicA, we are among addicts who get it,
who support each other in our recovery.
—Nicotine Anonymous Member

It was a tough struggle when I was being pulled on one side by addiction and the other side by the hope of freedom. The mental side of the struggle got me deeper into the addiction as I battled its insidiousness. My thinking had no effect on my ability to quit, because my intellect got blindsided by addiction and could not reason things out.

There is no logic to addiction, except that craving is simply withdrawal from the drug. Now I see the mind games I played to justify giving into the cravings and using nicotine to ease the withdrawal.

Boredom, ecstasy, sadness, stress, happiness, finishing a big project or starting one, fear, joy, luck, tragedy, fun, you name it, I smoked over it. It made sense at the time, until I began using the Tools of the program. And then, the denial lost its power, and I stood exposed to the sunlight of the spirit.

My friends in NicA showed me the actions that could change my thinking slowly over time, like attending meetings, working the Steps, doing service work, reading literature, reaching out, and practicing new behaviors. Taking these actions has changed my life.

*Today, I unshackle the chains of addiction
and step from slavery to nicotine into the miracle of freedom.*

JULY 19

Behind every fear, there is a miracle waiting to happen.
—Marianne Williamson

For 27 years, when I experienced anything that was emotionally upsetting, I would use nicotine to cope. The worst part of this was that, most of the time, what I was upset about would wind up easily working itself out.

The last 17 years of my active addiction, I tried to quit time and time again, and it seemed like nothing would ever work. I would get a few hours or days together, something would upset me, and I would use nicotine again. The shame, guilt, and remorse would get even worse when the situation would work itself out, but I had started my addiction all over again.

Now I relish the freedom of experiencing life without nicotine, and I know there are many ways of engaging in life other than using. I call someone in the program, go to an extra meeting, do Step work, or give service in the program.

When life works itself out, I don't have any shame or guilt. I use the program, not nicotine, to handle my emotions. I humbly accept the miracle that I get to feel the more uplifting emotions too, like joy, contentment, and the sweetness of life.

Today, I have options for how I respond to life's situations, and I choose to feel good.

JULY 20

I have tried all kinds of remedies and always failed.
NicA has kept me off nicotine. I couldn't have done it alone.
—Nicotine Anonymous Member

I smoked into my forties. I couldn't imagine a day without nicotine. Denial kept me from facing what a lethal killer my addiction was. I had more fear about quitting cigarettes than I did from diseases they cause. What insanity!

The grand hoax tells me I can't live without nicotine, an addictive substance which will cause a slow, miserable, painful death.

I had prayed for many years on and off for willingness, and it finally came. When I was ready, the miracle was there. I could finally say, "No matter what, I won't pick up." God was with me every step of the way. God held me and gave me strength. I am finally free.

Today, I am willing to go to any length to not light up.

JULY 21

Whatever you hold in contempt is your jailer.
—Brendan Francis

In order to recover from my addiction to nicotine, I did a searching and fearless moral inventory of myself. I uncovered my attitude of contempt towards others and even myself.

Contempt is defined as the feeling that a person or a thing is beneath consideration or worthless. Contempt is an attitude I expose to the sunlight of the spirit and become willing to have lifted.

When my anger is not resolved, it can remain stuck in contempt. Whenever my feelings become stuffed or stuck, I jeopardize my recovery.

Contempt is also an artificial way to feel better about myself by putting someone else down. Besides, whatever I protest about in another is usually a trait I overlook in myself. In recovery, I learn to hold my attitudes up like a mirror and keep the focus on my own shortcomings.

Contempt is a cold and empty place. My recovery will not grow there. Contempt separates me from healing. Recovery connects me with others in ways that are healing as we support each other. The Steps ask me to work humbly at my tasks. I am to think neither better nor less of another person. While contempt locks me in bondage, humility sets me free.

Today, my contempt is lifted, I am free to fulfill a higher purpose.

The community stagnates without the impulse of the individual.
The impulse dies away without the sympathy of the community.
—William James

One of the deepest human desires is to feel at ease with our connection to our community. The ease of that relationship depends upon mutual understanding and trust. At my first Nicotine Anonymous meeting, I was nervous and wary. As I listened to the welcoming introduction, I began to relax. When it was explained there was not to be any cross-talk, criticism, or unsolicited advice, I was relieved.

Although at first I did not fully understand the Twelve Steps and Twelve Traditions, I understood that the program had a path and a structure. It was powerful as members shared their experiences and extended their trust to the others. I felt that these people could understand my struggle with nicotine and my unease with living. The members' mutual support created a meaningful community that had been missing in my life.

Doing service has been the lifeline for my continuous recovery and has made me accountable to myself and to the community. I like the feeling of belonging and offering others mutual understanding and trust. I truly feel at ease.

Today, as my disease is lifted,
I am more at ease with myself and my recovery community.

JULY 23

While we are actively using
we cannot make our bodies stop craving nicotine,
but we *can* live with a craving until it passes...
—"Serenity Prayer for Nicotine Users"

Over and over I promised myself I would quit after the next pack, the next morning, after finishing a project, or on a big trip. Then a craving would come, and I couldn't handle the pain of withdrawal, so I lit up to ease the discomfort. Eventually, the discomfort of smoking became so painful that the withdrawal paled by comparison. I hit bottom in the misery of my powerlessness over this insidious addiction.

I found an online Nicotine Anonymous meeting of addicts who understood my torment. They showed me "The Serenity Prayer for Nicotine Users," which helped me learn about accepting that I'm going to crave as I withdraw from the drug. We discussed changing how we respond to the craving. I practiced the 5 Ds (Delay, Distract, Discuss, Drink water, Deep breathe), attended meetings, read NicA literature, worked the first two Steps with my sponsor, and began my conversation with my Higher Power. Finally, I set a quit date.

As a craving hit, I surrendered, and let the feelings wash over me. Going to any length to not light up became my mantra. The cravings eased over time. And soon the day came when I didn't even think about smoking.

Today, when a craving comes, I acknowledge and accept it.
I ask my Higher Power for help through the craving.
I go to any length to not light up.

Imagination was given to man to compensate him for what he isn't. A sense of humor was provided to console him for what he is.

—Horace Walpole

Left to my own experience as a nicotine addict, I couldn't imagine not using nicotine. I wished to be a non-user, but I couldn't see myself that way. For nearly three quarters of my lifetime, I had constantly used nicotine. When I heard and saw members share their recovery successes, I began to clear away the illusions of inadequacies that had limited my ability to even imagine being nicotine free.

I had considered myself a maverick, one who didn't go along with the flock. However, in my Nicotine Anonymous group, what I saw kept me returning each week. A member said that when she felt she couldn't show up due to her fears, she could act as if she was brave enough. She used her imagination to create the courage in herself that she didn't realize she had.

While working the Steps, I read, "Becoming humble was what it was all about." I found meetings had moments of comic relief when, even out of our madness and struggles, members could laugh at themselves. I laughed at myself too, humbled by seeing the humor of my own nonsensical behaviors. Letting go and acting as if, helped me imagine where I could be.

Today, I humbly imagine my wildest dreams with a grateful smile for how far I've come.

JULY 25

It is not the mountain we conquer but ourselves.
—Sir Edmund Hillary

For years, I thought my nicotine addiction was the mountain I had to conquer. Yet that task seemed too tall an order, too scary to attempt. I felt ill equipped, and I was, until I joined a Nicotine Anonymous group.

I found others who felt the same and those who had climbed the path to freedom. I learned NicA had Tools to equip members and had a path of Steps that other members had taken.

I witnessed others' progress as they followed our slogan, **Choose Faith Over Fear**. The longer I attended meetings, the more faith I had in the Steps. It became clear that there was more to change than my nicotine use. I needed to let go of my ineffective behaviors so that they could be lifted, so that I could engage in a more joyful life.

With the group's support and inspiration, I gained freedom. However, the main challenges remain: letting go of my old ways, continuing to practice new healthy behaviors, and practicing positive attitudes that are becoming my new normal. I have been given new Tools and equipment to keep climbing.

Today, I have faith that my shortcomings will be lifted,
as I take the Steps and use NicA's Tools.

JULY 26

Today is day nine, and I am having a complete meltdown.
—Nicotine Anonymous Member

For years, even the thought of withdrawal made me feel as though I was actually experiencing it. In hindsight, all that fear-based anticipation was like one long withdrawal. I had been alone and frozen in my fear. After months of NicA meetings, I finally took the desperate leap, borrowed just enough faith from my fellow members to let go, and tossed my last pack in the trash.

The initial days were rough, but not as bad as I had anticipated. I did not need to be confined for my own safety. By the end of the first week, I was beginning to feel a bit cocky, like I got this. That pink cloud turned to dark clouds soon after. I was in the midst of an emotional thunder and lightning storm. I was tossed and turned around every which way and had a complete meltdown. I was completely humbled.

Thankfully, I had a group phone list to call members as the storm raged on and off for the next few days. My friends in recovery got me through that challenge and others, as life's troubles came and went. Not only had I admitted I was powerless over nicotine, I fully experienced my powerlessness, as I held on to my fellow nicotine addicts and found safety and acceptance.

Today, I relax because I stay humble and connected to my meeting and its members, who inspire me to change.

JULY 27

The cravings would pass whether I indulged them or not.
—Sponsorship in Nicotine Anonymous (NicA)

When I first put nicotine down, I thought the cravings would never stop. I read "The Serenity Prayer for Nicotine Users" over and over. I discussed my cravings, did deep breathing, and drank lots of water. To distract myself and delay the cravings, I focused on tidying and cleaning to get my apartment in order.

When I got a year nicotine-free, my cravings had eased a great deal from the time I was a newcomer. I still used my phone list to reach out for support. At two years nicotine-free, my cravings were practically nonexistent.

I reach out to my sponsor when they happen. I still attend meetings regularly and serve on a Nicotine Anonymous committee to help carry out our primary purpose. I also reach out to newcomers. Using NicA's Tools of recovery is how I stay nicotine-free one day at a time.

Today, I am humbly grateful for the gifts of my recovery that have transformed my life.

JULY 28

As long as I was putting poison in my mouth,
my words were sending poison out of my mouth.
—Nicotine Anonymous Member

As a nicotine addict, the smoke I blew was filled with complaints. My negative thinking and behavior influenced me to have negative attitudes. Either I complained about whatever got in my way to use nicotine or I complained about myself, because I couldn't stop using nicotine.

A thorough Fourth Step helps me find those thoughts that create the under-my-breath grumblings. As I share my Fifth Step with my Higher Power and my sponsor, I experience a new kind of self- acceptance and grace. In my Sixth and Seventh Step, I work on dropping the negativity and changing my thinking.

In recovery, I have learned gratitude on a deeper level than my addiction had previously allowed. I am learning a new sense of sincerity as I experience fellowship. I am becoming more gracious with giving and receiving compliments. I allow others to help me in healthy ways. I am happier and feel a new generosity. It's as if a barrier has lifted. Most important, I am learning to love myself. I am grateful to my fellows for their support and acceptance.

Today, I have gratitude in my attitude.

JULY 29

Envy eats nothing but its own heart.
—German Proverb

As a child, I envied adults who could smoke. Smoking represented the power of privilege. I wanted to do what I wasn't allowed to do. As a teen, I started smoking because I envied cool and tough TV and movie stars who smoked. I continually compared myself to others. Was I better somehow, or worse? Envy eroded my self-esteem as it separated me from others.

When I first came to Nicotine Anonymous meetings, I was envious of those who had already gotten free of nicotine. I kept seeing them as better than me and myself as not enough, which didn't help me bond with the group.

However, I kept hearing that a principle of the program was to identify our similarities and avoid comparing ourselves to one another. When I identify with others, I connect with them. I let down my guard and relax—it's a good feeling. Comparing myself to others is a shortcoming I need to surrender, let go, and turn over. I am good enough just as I am.

Today, I add my envy to my inventory of traits that sever my connection to others.

JULY 30

The only requirement for Nicotine Anonymous membership
is a desire to stop using nicotine.
—Tradition Three

I love the way Tradition Three is so open and welcoming in spirit. Anyone can join Nicotine Anonymous with only the desire to stop using nicotine, regardless of their status of nicotine use or any other trait. Even if we just have a slight desire to get nicotine free, we will not be turned away. This program is here to help all nicotine addicts. We may have different opinions, and we might not take all suggestions that are offered to gain freedom from nicotine, yet we are still welcome.

I have heard it said to **Keep Showing Up**. Some may find their nicotine freedom right away and others might struggle for a while. It does not matter what form of nicotine delivery we use, we are all still welcome.

Where else can we go to hear the experience, strength, and hope of other nicotine addicts in recovery? This is Tradition Five in action, which says our primary purpose is to help the still suffering nicotine addict. The newcomer is the lifeblood of the fellowship, and at meetings the newcomer is the most important person in the room. We can each seek and ask for the help we need, and we find freedom from nicotine through this spiritual program of recovery.

Today, I have the desire to stop using nicotine,
and welcome the still suffering addict to our meetings.

JULY 31

There came a time when the risk to remain tight in the bud
was more painful than the risk it took to blossom.
—Anaïs Nin

Step sections in *Nicotine Anonymous: The Book* often speak about how feelings of fear and inadequacy relate to our addiction, both in the addiction's initiation and its ongoing grip. Feeling afraid and not good enough are paralyzing forces that once kept me stuck.

I'm grateful the only requirement for Nicotine Anonymous membership is a desire to stop using nicotine. I had long had that desire; it was my bud waiting to bloom. I had potential, but my feelings of fear and inadequacy kept me wrapped tight, unwilling to unfold.

My friends were nicotine users, and when I was alone those hits of nicotine were my friends. I believed they consoled me, my consolation prize for existing. I felt I deserved, at least, to have my nicotine for companionship.

I brought my bud of desire to weekly NicA meetings. Despite my doubts and fears, I followed our slogan, **Keep Showing Up**. I heard others share about reaching bottom. And they said, "I'm sick and tired of being sick and tired." Like them, I was desperate and stuck until our meetings gave me the willingness to let go, and let the program's powerful nurturing strength open the bud of my desire to quit, and blossom into a beautiful freedom.

Today, I tend to my recovery
in my garden of spiritual nourishment.

AUGUST 1

Made a list of all persons we had harmed,
and became willing to make amends to them all.
—Step Eight

My initial reaction to hearing this Step was avoidance. I did not want to re-experience the shame and other disturbing emotions related to my past behavior. However, *Nicotine Anonymous: The Book* says, "The purpose of this Step is to achieve freedom from guilt over our past actions and interactions with other people." I didn't get it. My way of achieving so-called freedom from such emotions had been to numb myself with nicotine, sucking those feelings deep down into my gut.

Eventually, meetings, literature, and my sponsor helped me realize the path to true freedom and peace. It was gut-wrenching coming to terms with the fact that I needed to face my past behaviors if I was ever going to relieve those feelings buried in my gut. If I kept them buried, I risked using nicotine again.

Step Eight is a simple part of the process of this gentle program; first just making a list and becoming willing. The principle of one day at a time is the same for one Step at a time, one increment of willingness at a time. This helps me manage what had once been unmanageable. My willingness is increasing as I make progress with my spiritual awakening.

Today, I come clean to heal my life in relation to others.

AUGUST 2

Forgiveness says you are given another chance
to make a new beginning.
—Desmond Tutu

I increasingly rely on the recovery principle of forgiveness. Forgiving others helps me let go of resentments and releases the debt. When I fully forgive, I feel a peaceful acceptance, a renewed sense of hope, and a new beginning.

Often, forgiving myself is much more difficult. Yet forgiving myself is a necessary component in my recovery and my everyday life. If I am unable or unwilling to forgive myself, I end up wallowing in the guilt, shame, and self-pity, which are the perfect recipe for a relapse.

In whatever ways I have practiced my defenses and defects of character, I take responsibility and make amends. I change the things I can, which are my own behavior, my thoughts and actions. As a spiritual being having a human experience, I make mistakes, as do others. With forgiveness of myself and others, I let go of what no longer serves me, and I am free to grow into the person I want to become.

In order to stay nicotine-free, I need that new beginning every day.

Today, I add myself to my amends list and become willing to forgive, change, and realize a new freedom.

AUGUST 3

There's a mental disconnect between my actions
and their consequences.
—Nicotine Anonymous Member

In active nicotine addiction, I felt the discomfort and fear of facing what I was doing. I disconnected my mind from the consequences of my behavior. I was unplugged. My addiction impacted my own life and the lives of those around me, especially those I loved.

I injured my health, and there were many things I didn't do or try which I could have enjoyed or valued, such as sports, jobs, and relationships. I excused or dismissed so many important aspects of my life. I polluted other people's air and landscapes, contributed to their illnesses, and set bad examples to their children.

Now, working Steps Eight, I am listing them all in preparation for making amends and changes. I am reconnecting my actions with their consequences. This is the continuation of cleaning up my life, which I started in Steps Four and Five. I am improving my contact with my Higher Power in order to make conscious decisions and practice NicA principles in all my affairs. What I do and think matters to me and those I'm connected to. Making responsible decisions plugs me into an energy source that improves my self-esteem and keeps me in a Good Orderly Direction.

---

*Today, I continue to take the Steps to a higher level
and prepare for the liberating Steps ahead.*

AUGUST 4

Rather than say I need to *work* on myself,
I say I need to *care* for myself.
—Nicotine Anonymous Member

Although it's my responsibility and requires effort, calling my recovery efforts *work* triggers my resistance reaction. In order to heal my disease, my sponsor suggested I consider following the Twelve Steps and program principles in all my affairs as a way to apply self-care. In Nicotine Anonymous literature, I read, "The power we actually want is love." And care is love in action.

From the time of my youth's bamboozled mind, I'd thought that using nicotine comforted me and was my caring companion. At least, that is, until I realized it wasn't. That's when the battle began between my inner spiritual self and the addiction. Nicotine became a love-hate relationship. This battle was exhausting and agonizing. Since I hadn't developed better options, I continued to use nicotine to relieve myself of that agony. How insane!

The battle consumed much time and energy over many years. The struggle affected and infected other decisions I made about my daily activities and life plans. When I found NicA, the Steps gave me an orderly plan to heal my physical disease, my mental delusions, and my spiritual battle. Caring for myself and others is now a daily practice of mutual support. How loving!

Today, I ask my Higher Power to "show me the way of patience, tolerance, kindliness, and love."

Love and compassion are necessities, not luxuries.
Without them, humanity cannot survive.
—The Dalai Lama

When I saw the announcement of a Nicotine Anonymous meeting in the local paper, I felt an immediate jolt of hope in my heart. I had been quitting the use of nicotine since I was 16 years old, and had failed again, and again, and again.

As a newcomer, I was without hope that I could ever stay quit. I had proven that to myself so many times. Yet, by the grace of God, I found myself at a Nicotine Anonymous meeting surrounded by all the support I needed. I knew that Twelve Step programs really worked. Another Twelve Step program had already saved my life. And now I had a program to free me from nicotine.

Even after joining NicA, I had a couple of slips. I listened to the members share how they succeeded, but I struggled to forgive myself. I felt they were superior, and I was weak, a failure. But that's not what they thought or said to me.

The kindness and acceptance of the members reaffirmed my faith in the 12-Step process. My fellow nicotine addicts understood that this is an insidious, cunning, and baffling disease. I was a struggling nicotine addict seeking a deeper level of willingness and self-forgiveness. That acknowledgement was the next right step in the right direction.

Today, I am willing to continue my healing process with courage and compassion.

AUGUST 6

If you want the real thing, you've got to sign up for it.
—Nicotine Anonymous Member

If I want recovery, I have to show up for it. I have to take reasonable risks. To become completely willing is to move beyond just wishing and wanting something better. I need to be willing to take the necessary Steps to get it.

In order to be authentic, I have to be present. I need to be front and center on my stage of life, not off in the wings. Yes, right there where others can see me, flaws and all. In order to have a life, I have to own it. To own it, I have to sign for it.

Recovery is about being responsible and accountable for my behavior in the here and now. I work the Eighth and Ninth Steps to help clean up my past harmful actions. I use the Tenth Step to keep clean in the here and now. Practicing the Eleventh Step helps to guide me as my days unfold.

When my efforts are continuous, sincere, and timely, I keep my life clean and my intentions clear for the real things to grow and flourish. And sometimes I have to get down on my knees and ask for guidance.

Recovery is a gift that arrives by spiritual delivery, but I still need to commit and sign my name to receive the delivery, the spiritual awakening in Step Twelve.

Today, I am responsible for my actions
as I take Steps through my day.

One meets his destiny often in the
road he takes to avoid it.
—French Proverb

Whether or not I was consciously trying to avoid feeling or dealing with situations in my life by using nicotine, I was. Nicotine had that effect. If avoidance was my goal, then using nicotine was successful. I thought I was controlling and directing my life. This made it difficult for me to admit how nicotine had made my life unmanageable and harmful.

Eventually my avoidance drove me down a road into a swamp of chaos. I needed NicA's know HOW to find serenity, peace, and even joy: Honesty, Openness, and Willingness. Fortunately, there was a NicA meeting nearby.

I have come to realize that in order to achieve freedom from my past behaviors and become the person I really want to be, I will have to do the Step work I have been avoiding. No matter which road I take, I end up where I need to be willing to face feelings and situations in my life with integrity. I now have the fellowship's guidance and support to help me on my daily journey.

Working the Steps is a way of addressing my former avoidances. I no longer want to look for detours, so I'll trust the path of progress I see in our program.

Today, I will follow our program's map,
because I can see fellow members up ahead.

AUGUST 8

Forgiveness is for yourself because it frees you.
It lets you out of that prison you put yourself in.
—Louise L. Hay

I'm always dazzled by what happens if I just wait to respond or to act. First, I want to get peaceful in my heart about the next right thing. If I stop and listen, take a short break, usually my Higher Power sends a thought, an invitation, or even a cool breeze or special token.

When my dearest friend said something that cut me deeply, I realized it was his issue and not my problem. I had to walk away rather than react with a sudden flurry of emotion. At home, I found my very special rock. This rock has marvelous stripes through it, one of which was split apart and then reattached with glue. You can barely tell, but I knew the story behind it.

I slipped it into my pocket, grateful for the imperfection of its fabulous beauty. It became my forgiveness rock. I held onto it all day, remembering that I forgive the rock for being broken, mended and healing, but still having its exquisite beauty.

In the same spirit, I can forgive my dearest friend with all his imperfections and broken places. I know his deep-down inner beauty. Like the forgiveness rock, he has stories behind those hurting wounds, just as I have mine. Acceptance of myself and others connects willingness to forgiveness.

Today, I forgive myself and others
for the imperfections and broken places,
and still love the beauty within.

AUGUST 9

The way not to lose heart is to realize
how everything we do matters.
—Pema Chodron

When I was smoking, I used to think that it didn't matter since I was only hurting myself. Now that I have some clean time, I realize I did harm, and that my smoking did matter. It mattered to my family and friends, it mattered to my physical and spiritual health, and it mattered that I was destroying life, even if it was my own. Knowing that my behavior does matter makes my life much more meaningful.

I no longer intentionally hurt myself. I take time to listen to what's really going on inside, to listen in meetings, and to listen for knowledge of my Higher Power's will for me. My life is a sacred gift from a divine source, and my work is to live it fully. My life matters.

Recovery is showing me the way of patience, tolerance, kindliness and love. It matters how I treat myself and others.

---

*Today, I ask myself, "Does it matter?" before I do something
that may harm others or jeopardize my serenity and my freedom.*

AUGUST 10

Pain nourishes courage.
You can't be brave if you've only had
wonderful things happen to you.
—Mary Tyler Moore

I have learned about myself that I only try to make a change if pain motivates me to do so. The pain of dying made me search out recovery. The pain of quitting led me to enjoy being a nonsmoker. The pain of the obsession to smoke gave me the courage to work the Steps, which lifted the obsession.

The first year of being off nicotine was a hard walk. I did not like it at the time, but as I look back on it now, the relief of living a nicotine-free life has stayed with me. I never want to go through that hard walk again. This motivates me to keep attending meetings, and to not forget the pain I would feel again if I was to go back to using.

I have to work at recovery to stay clean. When things are going wonderfully, and the sun shines down on me, and everything I touch turns to gold, I may risk forgetting the lessons I have learned. Although change can involve pain, the rewards of living happy, joyous, and free far outweigh any temporary discomfort.

*Today, I am willing to continue working the Steps,
even when it is uncomfortable.*

AUGUST 11

There is no one way for sponsorship,
only that which each member finds works for them.
—Sponsorship in Nicotine Anonymous (NicA).

My original home group's members didn't ask for or offer to be a sponsor. That Tool seemed more challenging for those unfamiliar with it than simply using the phone between meetings.

I used the *Nicotine Anonymous Step Study Workbook* to start taking that daring look deep into the mirror. The mirror revealed I had amends to make for some shameful acts in my past. I felt conflicted between wanting help and being afraid to expose my secret shame to a sponsor.

I moved and started attending phone meetings. There, I heard about NicA's booklet, *Sponsorship in Nicotine Anonymous.* I read the members' shares and got a better understanding of the mutual trust I could develop with a sponsor. I found a sponsor and together we determined how our relationship would work best for us.

As I've moved through this entire recovery process using the Tools, I've been willing to identify to whom and how my amends will be made. I'm building trust in myself and sponsorship. I'm experiencing a true healing beyond gaining freedom from nicotine. As promised, I'm beginning to love myself and continue to ask my Higher Power to do for me what I could not do for myself.

Today, I do my regular check-in with my sponsor
in order to remain honest, open, and willing.

AUGUST 12

You've been criticizing yourself for years and it hasn't worked.
Try approving of yourself and see what happens.
—Louise L. Hay

Growing up I learned to be hard on myself when I wasn't perfect in my thinking or behavior. I used this as a survival technique when faced with the wrath of my parents, because I so badly wanted my parents' unconditional love and acceptance. If I felt bad enough, they might feel sorry for me, and love me because I try so hard to be good and to be perfect.

Smoking helped me stuff back down those feelings of inadequacy, and in turn, I was harder on myself when I could not quit. I beat myself up over the many failed attempts to quit. The addiction was like a snake eating its tail in an endless cycle of quitting, failing, blaming, and shaming. It took surrendering to a Power greater than myself to finally end the cycle, get a quit going, and stop the self-destruction.

Learning to love myself, I practice self-compassion whenever I make a mistake. I forgive myself immediately, knowing I am a spiritual being having a human experience. Whenever I hear that old voice of shame and blame beating me down, I stop, stand up, brush myself off, and take three long, deep breaths. I return to my center of serenity, and acknowledge the whirling angst, let it go, and move onto a better feeling thought.

Today, Higher Power, please help me be kind to myself and treat myself with tender loving care, as you do.

AUGUST 13

Accept—then act. Whatever the present moment contains,
accept it as if you had chosen it.
Always work with it, not against it…
This will miraculously transform your whole life.
—Elkhart Tolle

The spiritual principle of acceptance has changed my life. When in active addiction to nicotine, I would fantasize that my life was different because I was afraid to face reality. This wishful thinking fed my addiction.

I now have a whole fellowship and a Higher Power to help me get free from fantasy and fear, to face life and not withdraw from it in denial of reality.

I denied the adverse effects of nicotine use. I told myself that fatal diseases associated with smoking may happen to others, but not me. Then I got an upper respiratory infection, and my doctor said I had early-stage emphysema. I still smoked, living in denial. The doctor must be wrong!

When I found Nicotine Anonymous, I was told I have a disease that tells me I don't have a disease. First, I admitted I was addicted to nicotine. Then, I found acceptance, just for this day, to live life on life's terms.

Acceptance is not always easy, especially after living in denial for so long. Whatever the circumstance, once I come to rest with it, I have many tools to help me live with the reality of the situation. I am grateful to this program, its Tools, and our fellowship for transforming my life.

Today, I accept the consequences of my addiction and ask for the courage to change the things I can.

AUGUST 14

We begin to forget we had been nicotine users,
except at meetings.
—"Our Promises"

I only wanted to stop vaping, but believed it was impossible for me to quit. Our Nicotine Anonymous "Slogans" pamphlet states, "Your 'impossible' becomes our 'possible' as we each realize that, together, we change."

This WE fellowship eventually helped me to be willing to go one hour without vaping, followed by another hour and then many more. That changed the impossible to possible, and this quit has lasted for several years. I am ever grateful, but remain humble.

Once it seemed impossible to even stop thinking about nicotine. My first weeks of freedom still seemed to confirm that as truth. But with time, most days, I had no thoughts or desires to use nicotine. It was as if I had forgotten I had been an active nicotine addict, except at meetings. That forgetting was relief from the madness of harming myself.

And those words in "Our Promises" were not just about enjoying the relief, but a reminder that attending meetings helps maintain our vigilance against relapse, lest we forget the power of nicotine and our powerlessness over it.

---

*Today, recovery is a verb, an ongoing process,
a truth to always remember.*

AUGUST 15

For me, there is no such thing as just one.
I cannot risk becoming complacent.
—*Year of Miracles*

My miracle happened due to my participation in and commitment to Nicotine Anonymous. I never quite understood why people stayed in the program for so many years after they had quit, although I was grateful they were there.

After eight years of being nicotine free I got complacent, and I stopped going to meetings, thinking that my addiction was gone. I thought I could use nicotine on my terms. I could not. I quickly found myself deep in a spiral of insanity and uncontrollability.

My addiction was not gone. My complacency had brought harm and shame upon my body and spirit again. I knew what I had to do. I came back to the program, and my miracle was there waiting for me, just where I left it. Members welcomed me and gave me just the support I needed to get free of nicotine again. I returned to my participation in and commitment to working my program, because this is what works for me.

---

*Today, I **Keep Showing Up**, because it works if I work it,
and we are all worth it.*

AUGUST 16

I came because of the smokes and stayed for the folks.
—Nicotine Anonymous Member

When I read *Nicotine Anonymous: The Book*, I identified with, "Deeply demoralized, we turned to Nicotine Anonymous as one more possible solution." Decades of nicotine use had me believe I couldn't live without those smokes, yet I knew they would kill me. Caught in that mental trap, I needed a solution, or at least a possibility.

I entered a Nicotine Anonymous meeting to stop smoking. I didn't know how and doubted anyone could actually help me. All I knew was that Twelve Step programs helped a friend recover from other kinds of substance abuse. I didn't know any specifics or whether I'd want to do anything involved in the program. I wasn't a club joiner. I didn't follow rules or like them.

Armed with my doubts and resistance, I entered the room. I was still smoking, but the members were welcoming and understanding. Those folks were awe-inspiring to me. They were why I kept showing up week after week. It would take time before I began to accept the program. It took months of their inspiration before I could finally let go of nicotine. I **Keep Showing Up**, because the members are one of my concepts of a Power greater than myself.

Today, as I enjoy clean time with my fellow NicA members,
I share and receive understanding, acceptance, and inspiration.

AUGUST 17

Be kind, for everyone you meet is fighting a harder battle.
—Ian Maclaren

When I'm around negative people and am unable to excuse myself to leave, often I recite the Serenity Prayer to myself as I listen and nod. If it's time for me to participate in the conversation or activity, I start with a statement of gratitude about something relevant. For example, "I am glad we get to discuss this..." or "Thank you for being here to work on this..." to defuse the negativity and get the focus back on some kind of positive perspective. It may take repetition to focus on the positive. Sometimes I must step back to protect my own serenity.

Often negative people are hurting; they act out because they don't know healthy ways to get relief from their pain. And so they take it out on others. I know that before recovery, that would have described me.

I learned recently that empathy is getting down into the other person's pain with them. Compassion is extending kindness, understanding, and a helping hand for one who is hurting to get up out of the pain. Those are principles for me to practice.

Today, I treat myself and others with patience,
tolerance, kindliness, and love.

AUGUST 18

When I vaped, I was lost in the clouds.
—Nicotine Anonymous Member

I started as a tough-guy-wannabe smoking unfiltered cigarettes. Later, I thought it wiser to model a cowboy by using filters. Years later, after a doctor's warning, I bought into ads for longer ultra-lights, believing they were safer. I only smoked more. My family begged me to quit. Eventually, with increasing health concerns, I switched to vaping. I hoped the promotional hype was true about vaping being the ultimate safe way to have my nicotine without worry.

Actually, vaping just became my latest attempt to not face the truth. I was still an addict, still compulsively using, still wasting money, and still had no faith that I could manage without some method to use nicotine. Then, the news of vaping-related damage and deaths blew away my fantasy, hiding in the clouds of vapor, I remained shrouded in fear.

I found Nicotine Anonymous on the internet and joined online and phone meetings. I didn't vape while I listened to others speak. It was a start. I bought NicA literature, including the *Nicotine Anonymous: Step Study Workbook*. Once I committed myself to work the program, I was lifted free of the shrouds and restored to sanity. That was a gift of joy for me, and for my family who had suffered watching my addiction.

Today, I pray, "Free me from fantasy and fear.
Inspire and direct my thinking today."

AUGUST 19

You can have a meeting without me,
but I can't have a meeting without you.
—Nicotine Anonymous Member

Since joining my original home group, I have been grateful to fellow members who show up each week. Then I moved and helped start a new meeting, and have been able to continually have a safe place to experience mutual support. Members from this group have helped to establish three other groups within driving distance.

Much of what is good in my life is a direct result of showing up at these meetings. They maintain my connection to fellow members and welcome newcomers. Meetings are a haven to heal the harms caused by our addiction. Because I know of people seeking local meetings where none currently exist, I do not take my meetings for granted.

Although resources from World Services are vitally important, my local members are absolutely essential. Their attendance and shares are the real, live inspirations that have kept me on course and Honest, Open, and Willing. That's HOW my recovery journey works.

Today, I have the willingness to ***Keep Showing Up***
and share this journey with my fellow members.

AUGUST 20

I've got to lighten up, instead of lighting up.
—Nicotine Anonymous Member

When I finally got serious about ending my use of nicotine, I searched and found Nicotine Anonymous. I was only vaguely familiar with 12-Step programs and not sure of what to expect.

Upon hearing the Twelve Steps read aloud, they sounded more than serious, even a bit morbid. There were those middle Steps all about "fearless moral inventory," "our wrongs," "our character defects," "our shortcomings," and "all persons we had harmed." I was already filled with shame and wondered whether this was time for my punishment.

But, I received such a warm welcome and was told that NicA was a gentle program of mutual support, and to go at my own pace. I could take what I want and leave the rest. That helped me relax. Each week we read one of the sections on the Steps. I learned I could also balance my inventory with my good qualities and assets. By acknowledging the people I had harmed, I was getting more honest and courageous. I became encouraged that the result of these Steps was a spiritual awakening. I wanted to be happy, joyous, and free. What relief! "Our Promises" really do come true.

Today, I remain serious about my recovery,
as I lighten up and relax.

AUGUST 21

One moment of patience may ward off great disaster.
One moment of impatience may ruin a whole life.
—Chinese proverb

When I was in the grips of my addiction to nicotine, I would usually react impulsively to everything. Typically, I would harm myself or others. I would have regrets about making rash decisions, and I would start craving nicotine. This continuous reactive behavior added to the endless cycle of my addiction and even more amends to make, and lengthened the list of those I had harmed.

I have learned through my experience with Nicotine Anonymous that it is wise to be patient. Now, I pause, wait and consider an appropriate response to any challenging situation. As I practice this new behavior, I develop more confidence in my decision making. I realize that my impatience in any situation or decision can risk a relapse or harm to myself or others. I maintain vigilance in order to respond in a healthy manner, so as not to jeopardize the joy of my freedom from nicotine.

Today, I continuously remind myself that patience can help restore me to sanity.

AUGUST 22

As life offers change moment by moment,
we are faced with a choice between faith and fear.
—Nicotine Anonymous "Slogans" pamphlet

After being overwhelmed with feelings focused on all that he was missing, my sponsee finally called and said, "I was suffering, but kept putting off calling you." Then he remarked, "That's like jumping off a bridge and planning to call after I hit the water." With his few months of nicotine abstinence happening in tandem with a global health crisis, his sense of loss and grief felt overwhelming to him.

Our program of mutual support asks us, both sponsors and sponsees, to learn from one another and how best to manage the constant changes in our lives. My lifetime is limited, so I need to use the Tools and spiritual guidance to lessen suffering. Using nicotine or my shortcomings are not solutions. Instead, I listen for the wisdom to do the next right thing.

Faith helps me manage change, and to find balance between loss and what I still have. I look for any possible benefits gained as the result of life's changes. Recovery has shown me that obstacles can sometimes lead to creative innovations and improved conditions.

Today, I am grateful I have resources to manage life's changes.

AUGUST 23

As smoking is to the lungs, resentment is to the soul,
even one puff is bad for you.
—Elizabeth Gilbert

When I stop to consider what my major triggers are, I realize that resentment is at the top of the list. Whether it's obsessing about what someone said or did, or wallowing in self-pity because the world isn't treating me fairly, resentment can ultimately lead to picking up again.

This realization has caused me to be much more conscious of my attitudes and their consequences for myself and others. I am realizing when it is just my shortcomings talking to me, and I question whether whatever I am feeling is really worth picking up over. When I get that familiar feeling of resentment taking my heart and mind into custody, I remind myself that resentment is bad for my soul and has harmed my relationships in the past. Resentments keep me from the peace that I seek.

Acceptance brings the peace I desire. If I let go of the outcome of a personal interaction or situation, I am free to feel serenity. The only thing I can control is myself and my response to people, places, and things. So, I work to accept the things I cannot change, which is everyone and everything else.

---

*Today, I accept what I cannot change
and change the things I can, myself.*

AUGUST 24

Some of us found it valuable to place ourselves
on our amends list.

—Nicotine Anonymous: The Book

I ask myself, in what ways am I keeping myself from completely and totally loving myself? What can I do to clear the way? Quitting nicotine has been the number one thing I could ever do to find an opening.

Early in my quit, the toxins were leaving my body and everything in my world was whacko for a bit. I was told to be extra tender with myself, take a nap, pause for an enjoyable moment, treat myself.

For me, quitting nicotine has been an emotional roller coaster at times. Other times, it's been like being a bull in a china shop; I have felt both clumsy and a bit fragile and breakable. And then there's being spacey, especially at first. Often I can laugh at myself and see ol' nicodemon's ruse to keep me totally distracted from being present in this moment, and from enjoying what's going on around me, and simply being content.

I've got to want this quit badly. It has had to be top priority, because I am healing from a disease caused by addiction. The great thing is, we are a fellowship of people who are going through this together, offering each other unconditional acceptance and support. By practicing what I am learning from my group, I am clearing the way for self-acceptance, self-appreciation, and truly loving myself.

Today, I clear the way for more love
and acceptance in my daily life.

We looked at the subtle harm we may have caused
in our relationships by the ways we had used cigarettes
as a barrier to intimacy, creating a smokescreen
to maintain an emotional distance
between us and those in our lives.
—Nicotine Anonymous: The Book

In Step Eight, I faced the harm I caused others which was a painful revelation. It meant taking a deeper look at the consequences of my addiction and adding many more people to my amends list. I knew about secondhand smoke, the offensive smell, the spilled ashtrays, and all the obvious harms I did to others. Now I was faced with acknowledging what might be considered the invisible harm I had not considered.

Did I really not know I used nicotine as an emotional hideout? Was it that I didn't want to admit it? While listening at meetings I came to realize I used smoking and nicotine to cover up my feelings of inadequacy. This started as a teenager, but never really ended. Using nicotine in this way also prevented me from improving interpersonal skills as I aged. Intimacy requires vulnerability, which can often be uncomfortable to someone who feels inadequate.

With this new perspective, I am having clearer insights. I better understand the consequences of nicotine to my past relationships. I wasn't fully present. There was a barrier, an underlying fear of exposing my inadequacies—my humanity. No wonder each new relationship was not all it might have been, yet expecting different results.

Today, I ask for the serenity to accept my past without shame, courage to live intimately, and the wisdom to know the difference.

AUGUST 26

Joy does not simply happen to us.
We have to choose joy
and keep choosing it every day.
—Henri Nouwen

The choices that I have each day are a product of praying to the God of my understanding to do God's will. As I work my program of recovery, I have faith and hope that one day I can bring joy into my heart. Even in the midst of pain, I can still experience joy.

When I slip into negative thinking, I let fear enter my mind and tell me that everything is hopeless. I do myself harm. Thankfully, the fellowship of Nicotine Anonymous supports me, and my sponsor offers thoughts of hope and encouragement. I use prayer and quiet time with literature and writing, which eases me into a state of freedom and joy.

When issues fester to the point of resentment, I take action. I share at meetings and with my sponsors about the issue. Once again, I am offered hope. I continue to take action and the issue resolves quickly. My serenity is mostly intact throughout the crisis, because I practice listening for my HP's will and asking for the support I need to continue to choose freedom and joy.

Today, I choose the freedom and joy promised in working the program.

AUGUST 27

Self-care is really about taking care of you and
focusing on feeling good about yourself—mind and body.
—Franchesca Ramsey

A member shared what her meeting experience meant to her: "For one hour, to pause, let go, and take in care for myself." For me, meetings are a safe haven during my week.

The first few months at meetings meant I had an hour when I didn't use nicotine. Meetings provided a pause in my madness. I could let go, and take in the care and encouragement from my fellow members. As a newcomer to Nicotine Anonymous, I was a nomad who had found an oasis in the midst of my desert of despair. I was welcomed and accepted. It was a refreshing respite from my own self-loathing.

Over the years, I've been focusing on Nicotine Anonymous rather than nicotine. Meetings are still a place of respite where I take in a lot of care. Increasingly, meetings offer an opportunity to give back and pay forward the wealth of wisdom I have heard—wisdom that helped me get free, stay free, and changed the direction of my life.

Sponsoring other members provides a purpose that helps heal the scars of addiction, both mine and theirs. Now, I'm less of a wandering nomad and more of a fellow traveler with a meaningful mission to care for myself and serve the fellowship.

---

*Today, I **Keep Showing Up** to welcome the newcomer
who seeks the same care and peace that I seek.*

AUGUST 28

At meetings, am I looking for help to step toward freedom,
or just for an audience to hear my woes of why I stay stuck?
—Nicotine Anonymous Member

The NicA meeting I joined ended with everyone saying, "It works if you work it, so work it, you're worth it." There's work involved? Of the shortcomings I would come to admit as a nicotine addict, I didn't really want to have to work, or wait. I was quite accustomed to having relief and satisfaction within seconds; it was quick and easy, if I let denial cover up the reality of what I was doing to myself.

Denial's backup was a long list of excuses for how and why I used nicotine. I had complaints and grievances about my life's situations. At first, the meeting seemed the ideal place to have them all heard. I could back up my truck of troubles and dump them on the table and then go home and use nicotine. I got some emotional relief, but I didn't get recovery. I was still stuck.

Frustrated, I got a sponsor. My sponsor explained meetings are mainly a place for our mutual support by sharing what each is doing to recover. Simply dumping my woes was just about me, and not about we. My sponsor was willing to hear my struggles, but to get unstuck, I then needed to commit to doing the work to moving forward.

Today, I accept that progress comes when I commit to using the Steps and Tools, because I'm worth it.

Cries for help are frequently inaudible.
—Tom Robbins

My life was like a pendulum swinging all over the place, and no matter what I did or where I was, my one constant in the chaos was a hit of nicotine. I was never without one.

I had quit before, but that was a bust after thirteen days because I had no support. When I got COPD, I was desperate to get quit once and for all, so I went to any means possible to find a way to get free and stay free from nicotine. Reaching out for help was difficult. Hadn't I handled all the chaos myself? And yet there was that wee small voice crying so loudly for help.

I was introduced to Nicotine Anonymous by both my therapist and my desperation to find relief; for this I am grateful. The meetings truly saved my life. Now I am nicotine free, and I am humbly grateful.

Today, I am no longer in a dark hole filled with quicksand, now I've got a flashlight and friends to help me out.

AUGUST 30

I have found that if you love life, life will love you back.
—Arthur Rubinstein

Today I focus on loving myself and loving life. Loving myself emotionally, mentally, and spiritually, I forgive and accept myself exactly as I am and I repeat positive affirmations about myself and life. When my thoughts are positive, I love life. Then the whole world opens up to me as I open up to the world.

I receive love by giving it. And as I reach out and help others, love is returned exponentially. To help another who has a similar addiction or compulsion, I reach out and share my experience, strength, and hope in gratitude for my nicotine freedom. *You can't keep it unless you give it away.*

Now I can say I love life, even though life is not going entirely how I think it should. I am growing, my physical health is improving, and by using the Tools of the program, I get unstuck and do the next right thing to love myself and life.

Finally, after decades of smoking that kept me stuck doing the same harmful things over and over, I can now choose to love myself, love life, and see my life continually getting better.

Today, I change my thinking by taking action toward loving myself and loving life.

AUGUST 31

Our purpose was not to evaluate the behavior of others
but to look only at our part of the interaction.
—Nicotine Anonymous: The Book

There is powerful wisdom in the Step Eight section of *Nicotine Anonymous: The Book*. Working this Step was a challenge for me. I had mostly evaluated hurtful interactions by weighing who was most at fault or justifying my part because of another's actions. By now, I have begun to realize how unmanageable or unproductive that weighing method was. It just weighed me down. It wasn't solution-focused or achieving the peace that I seek.

If I am to live a clean, nicotine-free life and remain restored to sanity, I need to live based on sound and sane principles. To be thorough in this effort *The Book* also guides me to admit the harm I did that was not directly related to my nicotine addiction. Nicotine stunted the growth of my emotional intelligence and impacted my relationships. I experienced great pleasure and deep pain in my relationships; they are essential and are the "We" of this fellowship.

It's a big Step to take responsibility and list all I've harmed in some manner. One day at a time, these Steps have brought me this far, so I will continue to trust them.

---

*Today, I am improving my interpersonal responses
by taking responsibility for my behavior.*

SEPTEMBER 1

Made direct amends to such people wherever possible,
except when to do so would injure them or others.
—Step Nine

For me, Step Nine has been the most difficult Step. With the previous Steps, I fluently wrote all the answers to the questions in the *Step Study Workbook*. I talked about them to my sponsor every week. I had experience with Step work in other programs, but in this program, I found it very difficult to make amends.

At Step Eight, I listed all persons I had harmed, including those I had harmed by lying. To the outside world, I lived a clean and healthy life while secretly, I was smoking. When life got difficult, I believed I needed to smoke.

I kept working on my list and sharing about it. I'd put it away, then work on it some more. I knew I had to move forward and make amends to everybody I lied to. So many people!

I'm doing Step Nine bit by bit, lovingly, kindly, making direct amends when possible, and indirect amends by contributing to a smoke-free world. My sponsor suggested I can be creative. I organized a breathing workshop and donated all benefits to a charity.

I don't have to do Step Nine perfectly or even all at once. I just have to take action and work at it one day at a time.

Today, I do the best I can. It's about progress, not perfection.

SEPTEMBER 2

Within the word "amend," its purpose is revealed—a mend.
—Nicotine Anonymous Member

By making amends I am seeking to make a mending in my life in order to heal wounds within myself and between myself and others. I say *Amen* to that!

However, when I first read Steps Eight and Nine, I thought I would feel more guilt and shame. Then I got a sponsor who pointed out there was a reason they were Steps Eight and Nine and not One and Two.

The Steps are an orderly process to address the chaos of my unmanageable life. First, I needed to get right with myself and do some self-mending. I worked Steps One through Nine to help me attain clarity, humility, and courage to mend myself and my relationships with others. Step Ten is there because I continually seek progress; I am not perfect.

I've done a lot of mending and there's a lot yet to do. It's an ongoing process of healing. I've let go of a lot of shame connected to my past. I now welcome making living amends with each day by my choices of behavior and attitudes.

Today, I am healing with my mending,
as I get right with myself and others.

SEPTEMBER 3

I am my own hero. First, I am kind to myself,
and second, I do things I want.
—Third Grader

This kid is my hero. Being kind to myself was a challenge when I was using nicotine. I was so desperate to avoid feeling anything by numbing my emotions with nicotine that I had no idea how to find comfort in healthy ways. I didn't know how to be kind, generous, and loving to myself. In recovery, I am learning how to be kind and make amends to myself by taking good care of my physical, emotional, and spiritual wellbeing.

Being kind to myself means avoiding toxic people and situations, and delegating responsibilities when my plate is overflowing. Being kind to me also means scheduling several hours each day for my own enjoyment and pleasure such as walking, preparing a nice meal, attending meetings, reading, doing service work, and having fun.

I had no idea what I wanted when I was using nicotine, other than to continue the cycle of addiction. In recovery, I am learning what I like and what I want, and how to stand up for myself while still being kind to myself and others.

Today, I am my own hero, and I am kind to myself and others.

SEPTEMBER 4

As long as you're feeling, you're healing.
—Nicotine Anonymous Member

When I was in active addiction, I spent all of my energy on smoking and isolating, smoking and isolating, smoking and quitting, quitting and smoking—a whirlwind of stress. I am grateful to not be active in this spiral of madness anymore. Now, I focus on being much more aware of my emotions and where I put my energy.

The beginning of my quit was rough because of the rawness of my emotions. I wasn't burying my feelings in a haze of nicotine anymore. I was learning how to feel again and what to do with those feelings.

Now, life isn't perfect, but it's better. I get to enjoy myself by doing fun activities like going on trips, playing sports, and other fun games. Why not try face painting, animal balloons, and dancing? I now have a chance to have amazing times and share the joy with others.

I am grateful for these opportunities to express my emotions in a healthy way as I let go of the past and make amends to myself. As my old wounds heal, I am grateful for the lessons. I no longer react in crazy ways to having emotions. Instead, I am learning to feel what arises and accept the feelings, regardless how uncomfortable. In acceptance, I find peace.

Today, I am grateful for the grace of this program, and my new ability to fully feel my feelings and accept them.

SEPTEMBER 5

We awaken in others the same attitude of mind
we hold toward them.
—Elbert Hubbard

Each time we engage with another person, we reflect in each other what we see in ourselves. We all like to be reassured that we are valued and accepted. We each seek connection with our true selves in each other's reflection.

We exist as individuals, and live as a community—each connected to and affecting the other. So, we each have a responsibility to reflect in each other the goodness we have awakened in ourselves. Today, I am responsible for my own healing and making amends to those I have harmed in the past.

Sharing in meetings is a powerful example of how each of us is a mirror for others. When I share my experience, strength, and hope, I hold these qualities up as a mirror. As I see my fellow members as sources of recovery, they can see those qualities in themselves. This is how we can awaken new attitudes that help each other move forward toward a new kind of freedom.

Today, my example and my opinion are powerful tools that create the kind of world I live in.

SEPTEMBER 6

I think one's feelings waste themselves in words;
they ought all to be distilled into actions
which bring results.
—Florence Nightingale

I treated feelings like facts. I felt the only way I could have relief was by using nicotine. Members of Nicotine Anonymous showed me that the only power and reality behind my feelings is what I grant them.

I experience an entire range of feelings from disturbing to ecstatic, and fearful to joyful. In fact, they are a stew of mixed emotions. I've learned that at any time I can reach down inside myself, into the stew, and pick out another emotion to focus on.

When I got the news that a family member died, I was very sad. The grief took over my emotions, yet I reached down and remembered the joy I felt because we had such a great relationship. And then I was able to see and feel my gratitude for my recovery. I am able to choose what I want to feel and still really feel my feelings.

When I was in early recovery from nicotine, I examined my isolation and decided to change that. I sought out long neglected friends and family. Some friends and family responded, some didn't. One dear cousin, Joy, welcomed me warmly. If I hadn't gotten clean, I would have missed Joy. Now I will always welcome joy in my heart. That's the kind of emotion I choose to feel.

Today, I focus on positive emotions
and feel the goodness of gratitude.

SEPTEMBER 7

Wellness seeks more than the absence of illness;
it searches for new levels of excellence.
—Greg Anderson

My philosophy was to quit using nicotine and deal with the rest later. I asked everyone around me for mercy and tenderness as I began recovery from this insidious addiction. And I treated myself with gentleness as the waves of cravings passed.

I gained weight because of the extra food and sugar intake. However, I did not light up while working through stressful situations. The fellowship suggests **The Weight Can Wait**, because getting free of nicotine is such an enormous undertaking.

It was the meetings, working the Steps with my sponsor, doing service work, reading, and reaching out to others that helped me get back to a more balanced lifestyle. As an amends to myself, I was eating well, sleeping well, being active, participating in NicA, and having a life. Over the many years I've been quit, I have lost the weight I gained, and gained some back, and am now losing some again. And so it goes as we age.

Some of us discover underlying health issues brought about by nicotine use, because nicotine can affect other aspects of our overall well-being aside from respiratory issues. Checking in with medical professionals for the help needed for quality of life is an important aspect of recovery. I am willing to go to any length for self-care.

Today, I ask for help to make the necessary changes in my lifestyle to include what's needed for my well-being.

SEPTEMBER 8

Recovery teaches us that our behavior and attitude are choices.
—Nicotine Anonymous "Slogans" pamphlet

When anxiety began to raise its ugly head, I might as well have been a movie script writer, as well as the projectionist. I could conjure up a whole disaster movie and project it into my future.

Over my lifetime, I wonder what percentage of these "disaster movies" have ever come close to resembling anything that actually happened to me. At this moment, I can't think of one. And as I wrote those scripts, how many times did I reach for yet another dose of nicotine thinking it was what I needed, that it would be my savior?

Now, NicA guides me to live morally right with hope, make amends, and stay grounded in gratitude for my freedom from nicotine. I never know what's around the corner, so there is no reason to give up and pick up. I've come to accept the NicA slogan, **Smoking is Not an Option** and the truth that nicotine will not solve a single problem. I've come to believe in a faith of my own understanding, which inspires me to act with courage and project positive possibilities.

Today, I use our wise slogans
to help me make good decisions.

SEPTEMBER 9

Even the smallest act of caring for another person
is like a drop of water—
it will make ripples throughout the entire pond.
—Jessy and Bryan Matteo

I am thinking about all of my friends in the program who have shared their experience, strength, and hope with me, and who helped me find my way. They loved me when I could not love myself. I began to trust them, because I felt I could not trust myself. I saw how my addiction robbed me of trust and love, and how my fellow NicA members' unconditional acceptance and support fed my strength to break the bonds of addiction.

As I worked the Steps, my relationship with my Higher Power grew, and I began to trust that the God of my understanding would be there for me just like my fellow addicts had been. And I began to trust myself. And as my trust grew, so did my love.

Thank you NicA for holding space for my recovery, and giving me hope. I can live a nicotine-free life, and be the very best I can be.

Today, whenever possible, I help others by showing my gratitude for what I have been so freely given.

SEPTEMBER 10

If we romance it, we chance it.

—Nicotine Anonymous "Slogans" pamphlet

For years I wrapped my life around feeding the lies of my nicotine addiction. Through this dishonesty with myself and others, I selfishly put smoking cigarettes above just about everything else in my life. I only dreamed of breaking free from the addiction; it was impossible to stay quit by myself.

After a long struggle trying to break free from the unending spiral of craving and using nicotine, I finally surrendered. I am nicotine-free through the Nicotine Anonymous meetings, literature, service, Steps, and reaching out to others. "Our Promises" talk about the "grand hoax," that "we have not given up anything at all." I understand this now that I am nicotine-free. What was the big attraction that prevented me from giving up nicotine?

I have heard it said the opposite of love is apathy. In stating that I have not given up anything at all, I'm embracing self-care. I don't *romance* cigarettes. I walk away with no regrets. I ask that all delusions of love for smoking be removed. I make amends to myself by replacing those delusions with loving self-care.

Today, I am honest with myself and others
as I let go of the fatal attraction to nicotine.

SEPTEMBER 11

Persistence and resilience only come
from having been given the chance
to work through difficult problems.
—Gever Tulley

When I feel I'm slipping down into my old darkness, my group lifts me up to realize a new resilience. How amazing that I'm getting through all these feelings without using nicotine replacements anymore. Sometimes I feel an overwhelming variety of uncomfortable and awful feelings: anger, rage, shame, longing, self-loathing, and despair.

When I'm in the throes of such discomfort, I often forget that a feeling will pass, just as a craving will pass whether I use nicotine or not. I struggle until I find the willingness to remember that feelings are not forever; and if I use nicotine even once more, I'll just start the cycle of addiction all over again.

I have worried about showing up at a meeting, and no one being there, because they all had gotten better and left. I fear that I would slip back into isolation and pick up nicotine, thinking that using the substance is the solution. That's when I have learned to pick up the phone instead, or get myself to the next available NicA meetings ASAP.

I am incredibly grateful for my fellow members' support. As I let cravings for nicotine and those uncomfortable feelings pass, I strengthen a new resilience. I believe I truly can amend my ways and be restored!

Today, with the mutual support of my fellow members,
I develop resilience and find an enduring faith
in being restored to sanity.

SEPTEMBER 12

We are learning to assert ourselves
where previously we have been aggressive or passive;
We are also beginning to love ourselves.
—"Our Promises"

When I was an active addict, I beat myself up constantly. No criticism that came from the outside world could possibly compare with my own inner critic. I said unkind, cruel, and hurtful things to myself throughout the day—things that I would never dare say to another person. No matter what I accomplished or how much progress I made, I told myself it was not good enough. No matter what circumstances I endured or how much effort I made, I hardly ever treated myself with compassion. Instead focused on how I should have done better.

In my recovery from nicotine addiction, I am learning how to love myself bit by bit, one day at a time. Slowly, thoughts of unworthiness are being replaced with feelings of acceptance and belonging. When I share my stories and struggles with other members, I often hear how what I have shared has helped them in their recovery. Knowing that I am helping others improves my self-esteem and provides me with a sense of purpose in my life. I am becoming someone I really like, thanks to the fellowship of Nicotine Anonymous.

Today, I forgive myself for the harsh ways
I have treated myself in the past,
and I open myself up to the compassionate,
unconditional love of my Higher Power.

There's no such thing as a problem
without a gift for you in its hands.
We choose these problems,
because we need their gifts.
—Richard Bach

Although nicotine is an insidious addiction, I am grateful for the opportunity to learn and grow in my recovery. The Twelve Steps are my guideposts for sanity and serenity for living life on life's terms, not nicotine's. No longer am I controlled by nicotine, imprisoned by the constant urge to use. No longer does my addiction lie to me about my self-worth.

As I've worked each Step, both my shortcomings and assets have been revealed. As I let go of the shame and guilt caused by my addiction, I can see that I am a good person. As I make amends, I forgive myself and others for the past, so that I can be fully present in this moment.

I celebrate my recovery as my new life is unfolding. I breathe in the good life I'm creating, and let go of old behaviors that no longer serve me. These are the gifts of recovery that I have needed for so long. I deserve to have a good life and to live joyfully.

Today, I am enough just as I am right now.

SEPTEMBER 14

When you find peace within yourself,
you become the kind of person
who can live at peace with others.
—Peace Pilgrim

During high school and college, smoking started out as a way to fit in with new friends and in new social situations. But as I got older, I isolated myself more and more to feed my nicotine addiction. I excused myself from meetings, meals, and other gatherings so that I could smoke. I always made sure I took my smoke break, whether or not anyone wanted to join me. I didn't care what I missed or who I may have offended as long as I got my fix. As time passed, I found myself feeling more lonely and less connected to those I cared about.

When I came to Nicotine Anonymous, I learned how to build healthy human connections again. As I listened to people share during meetings, and talked to members before and after the meetings, I realized I wasn't so alone in the world. I found other people out there who I could relate to. I no longer felt the need to escape conversations by running away to smoke. It felt good to make amends to myself and others for the ways I had sabotaged relationships. Slowly, I became more comfortable in my own skin, and found others who appreciated and loved me for being the unique individual I am.

Today, I express my gratitude for the fellowship
I have found in Nicotine Anonymous,
and for new ways of relating to others.

SEPTEMBER 15

I surrendered and now realize the power of Yes.
—Nicotine Anonymous Member

Several chapters in *Nicotine Anonymous: The Book* describe how fear and feelings of inadequacy are involved in our shortcomings. I sought out a chemical solution, but I caught an addiction. As a teen, I wanted to safely fit in, yet stand out within my peer group. Nicotine seemed able to block out fear and feelings of inadequacy.

Nicotine gave me the power of *No*. Blowing smoke said *No* to my parents' rules and to all uncomfortable feelings. I was even saying *No* by defying the health threats until a doctor said otherwise. After that, no amount of nicotine could block out the fear and feelings of inadequacy to stop my addiction.

My salvation began when I said *Yes* to join a NicA group, despite my doubts and fears. Next, I said *Yes* to service, despite wanting *No* responsibility. But it was finally the *Yes* when I had the gut-wrenching coming-to-terms that I was hooked on a drug, and that recovery is not a journey that one travels alone. *Yes*, I finally surrendered and experienced freedom by the power of *Yes* in this *WE* program.

Today, I make amends to myself by saying Yes to new possibilities.

SEPTEMBER 16

A well-developed sense of humor is the pole
that adds balance to your steps
as you walk the tightrope of life.
—William Arthur Ward

I don't know if all nicotine addicts are serious like me, but I have a lack of having fun and laughing during my active use of nicotine, and sometimes during my recovery too. My greatest problem is taking myself very seriously.

Addiction to nicotine is a serious matter. The facts point to the deadly nature of smoking, chewing, and vaping. The consequences of nicotine use are truly detrimental to us emotionally, mentally, and spiritually. The benefits of quitting are freedom, happiness, and joyous living.

It has been recommended to me to make amends to myself by making time for fun in my life. As a child, I didn't need this advice because I naturally knew how to enjoy fun and humor. Now in recovery, I am learning to see things as funny or humorous. I believe the God of my understanding has a sense of humor, especially when I take myself too seriously. This puts life in a new and enjoyable perspective.

Humor and fun activities are making my recovery much easier. Having fun relieves a lot of stress for me, and goes a long way toward living an enjoyable nicotine-free life.

---

*Today, I am discovering more ways to find the humor in life
and more activities that provide enjoyment and fun.*

Nothing changes if nothing changes.
—Hindu Saying

I was unsuccessful at quitting by cutting down on my smoking. It would work for a while, but eventually I would always go back to using as much as before. I needed to change. I needed NicA's help.

When I first put down nicotine, I missed the feeling of smoke going into my lungs. I replaced the sensation by using the tip to take deep breaths, which worked well for me. I got used to not moving my hand to mouth with other strategies. I frequently chewed on the end of a straw. Sometimes I chewed on carrots, nuts, or licorice. In the beginning of my quit, I used these strategies to help take the edge off cravings. I was able to delay and distract myself from reacting like I always had to when withdrawing from the drug.

My sponsor suggested getting rid of anything that was associated with smoking. I found it really helpful to throw out all of my addiction paraphernalia. I put anything associated with using nicotine as far away from me as I could.

To quit this addiction, I have had to change the way I behave and think. I can no longer believe every thought I think. But I can count on my breath, my Higher Power, and the fellowship to help me through.

Today, if I have the urge to smoke, I take a long deep breath and thank my Higher Power that I still have the ability to do so.

SEPTEMBER 18

This is a "We" Program
—"World Services, My Intergroup, and Me"

Nicotine use, for me, started as an attempt to connect to a peer group. However, my addiction to nicotine became a disease of disconnection and irresponsibility. I may have supported my addiction with my own money, but my behavior with nicotine, especially spreading secondhand smoke, was anything but responsible. Smoking was all about *my* need. I thought I cared about others, but my actions spoke louder than any sentiments. I have amends to make.

Tradition Seven guides us "to be fully self-supporting," which directly relates to my accepting responsibility. The word self, in this context, is not just about supporting me. I accept that we each are responsible for the fellowship's welfare, because my personal recovery depends on this unified support. The principle also connects me to all the members—the "We."

I demonstrate my amends by taking responsibility for contributing service and making regular monetary contributions to my group, Intergroup, and World Services. My ability to sustain myself physically, emotionally, and spiritually, both in and out of the fellowship, depends on doing my part to support Nicotine Anonymous, and not expecting others to do it for me.

Today, I am maturing into a responsible member
who supports the "We" program" that saved my life.

SEPTEMBER 19

If I can't handle not being good at something,
how could I consider myself a successful person?
—Gerald Hodges

I watched a story about Gerald, a top high school athlete, who couldn't swim. The swim coach needed another body on the swim team to compete. Gerald signed up and worked hard to learn to swim. This quote was his answer to why he took on the challenge, exposed his inabilities to schoolmates, until he improved by the end of the season to get the team to the state competition.

I didn't attempt to stop smoking during all the years I wanted to. This was, in part, because I couldn't handle not being good at something. I didn't want to feel the failure, nor have others watch me fail. Joining Nicotine Anonymous was the antidote to those fears. My meeting was my *school pool* to learn how to swim. I showed up weekly, failing to stop, but there was no judgment, no ridiculing, only support that kept me afloat.

I'm still swimming laps without nicotine. Based on that success, NicA has given me the courage to take on other challenges I wasn't good at. Now, I can more confidently handle the initial fears of failure. I know I have NicA's support. It's been my key to becoming a *successful person*.

Today, I ask yet again for the courage to keep improving my life.

SEPTEMBER 20

It's easier to fool people than to
convince them that they have been fooled.
—Mark Twain

Was that ever true when I was just a Huck Finn boy who escaped with stolen cigarettes or cigars into the woods to walk along the railroad tracks or up a stream. I grew up in a culture watching adults smoke and being mesmerized by movie scenes and billboard ads. I was a rebel without a clue. I wanted to identify with characters in those ads. They fooled me into believing using tobacco was the good life, both exciting and relaxing.

My Huck Finn was soon hooked on those ad lines and sinking into a deep addiction. I think getting away with stealing my parents' cigarettes or cigars was the beginning of my spree into crimes and misdemeanors during my young years. Not only had I been fooled about tobacco, but I fooled myself into thinking I was getting away with things just because I didn't get caught. It was the beginning of the grand hoax for me.

With adulthood came days of reckoning when I needed to convince myself that I had fooled myself. I hadn't really gotten away with anything, certainly not with using nicotine. A doctor's report was a rude awakening. Huck needed more than luck—he needed a program of recovery.

Today, I am grateful
I no longer participate in the grand hoax.

Now, we learned how to incorporate pleasure
into our lives in healthier ways.
—Nicotine Anonymous: The Book

For years, I knew I needed to *stop* smoking, but without any thoughts about what I needed to *start* doing. The chemical addiction and my repeated behaviors had me believe that nicotine served all my emotional needs. I even believed it was my best friend. Actually, it was merely my constant companion, especially when I felt lonely. I believed nicotine created my daily pleasures—to perk me up in the morning, give me pauses during the day, and soothe me in the evening. Yet, in moments of reality, my deteriorating health haunted me.

At meetings, I heard, "Nothing changes, if nothing changes." *The Nicotine Anonymous Newcomer's Booklet* says, "Action creates hope." I needed to insert healthy activities in my daily routine if I was ever to remove the toxin nicotine as a means to have my comfort and enjoyment needs met.

My sponsor suggested if I wasn't willing to stop using nicotine today, I could start incorporating healthy pleasures without delay. I was accepting the possibility of hope as I witnessed what other members did that worked for them. In the past, I had only wanted to *stop*, but now, I *start* being willing to participate in healthy self-care.

Today, I pause to create healthy pleasures for myself.

Most human beings have an almost infinite capacity
for taking things for granted.
—Aldous Huxley

When I transitioned from active addiction to my first weeks of abstinence, I shocked myself at having a thought that quitting smoking was no big deal. After some two decades of wanting this freedom, months of attending meetings, my brain has that thought? Oh, this cunning addiction would have me take this freedom for granted. How dangerous!

During the years since, I have observed members who were grateful for their freedom and those who appeared to take it for granted. There were those who faithfully utilized the entire program and those who chose to only use some of it. Although I appreciate that members can take what they want and leave the rest, I made a decision about what was best for me: to make a commitment to **Keep Showing Up** at meetings, practice NicA principles, and to accept my freedom as a sacred gift. It is a big deal and I want to keep it.

Today, I confirm my humble gratitude for this sacred gift and vow never to take it for granted.

SEPTEMBER 23

Having a happy and balanced approach is what I strive for,
otherwise, I make myself miserable.
I did that long enough!

—Nicotine Anonymous Member

I started out my quit chewing gum and sucking on mints. It was too much sugar, but it got me through some rough spots. I drank LOTS of water. At first, I gave myself permission to enjoy most anything (but nicotine), and gained some weight. I expected it, because I quit at Thanksgiving, but didn't beat myself up over it. I was just glad to be off the nicotine. I heard our slogan, **The Weight Can Wait**, and was tender with myself.

Then I discovered after all the years of smoking, my body had some deficiencies and went through some changes. I started really listening to my body and what I was really hungry for, such as protein in the mornings or strawberries in spring.

Thankfully, I love to walk, and so I walked and walked. My doggie was sure happy about that. I could use my body and actually breathe! And as I got active, the weight slowly began to come off.

I do splurge on a few yummy treats now and then. It's okay as long as I keep moving and eat other good stuff, like lots of fruits and veggies and whole clean foods. I've learned through this process to allow myself to enjoy food, so that I won't obsess.

Today, I enjoy a balanced and healthy lifestyle,
and that helps me to feel good and be happy.

There is nothing in the world so irresistibly contagious
as laughter and good humor.
—Charles Dickens

I had tried to quit smoking so many times it would have been difficult to keep track. Nothing worked. I truly believed that I was going to die as a nicotine addict, and I accepted that.

One day while laughing with my four-year-old daughter, I had to stop because my lungs hurt. She didn't understand why we had to stop playing. My addiction was not letting me live life. I dragged myself to a Nicotine Anonymous meeting and my miracle happened.

As soon as I began working the Steps, I was able to get a quit going. Then, as I learned more about myself and what I didn't want, I started choosing the kind of life I had always wanted. I found sweetness and humor in the joys of living life on life's terms. As my daughter grew, we have laughed ourselves silly many times.

I quit for me and as an amends to my daughter. The joy in that child's eyes continues to make my recovery a rewarding experience. Thank you Nicotine Anonymous, for giving me back my life.

Today, I enjoy laughter, love, and living this amazing life.

SEPTEMBER 25

It takes time to make amends.
We learned patience through the process.
—Nicotine Anonymous: The Book

In early recovery, I often asked myself how I would achieve living without nicotine over the long-term? A number of members in my NicA group had a lot of clean time. I looked at them with envy and awe. How did they do it? What's the secret? I got involved in the program. I worked the Steps and did service work. I lived life, and I stopped worrying about the secret.

Now, many years later, I have that once mysterious long-term freedom from nicotine. I see that the secret is actually no secret at all. It is given to me at every meeting as each member shares their experience, strength, and hope. It is laid out for me in the slogans, like **Keep Showing Up** and **Together We Change**. It is continuously modeled for me as I watch fellow members work the Steps and the Traditions.

The itch inside that told me I had to have a nic-fix was a lie. No amount of nicotine can heal what only a Higher Power can. Daily surrender to my own Higher Power is how I achieve long-term freedom from nicotine—one day at a time.

Today, I stay in the present, do the next right thing,
and leave the rest to my Higher Power.

That doesn't work for me.
—Charles Weatherby

I was having an earnest discussion with a loved one. I wanted him to do something my way. I don't remember now what it was that was so important. I do remember that each time I put forth a perfectly compelling argument, he said, "That doesn't work for me." I thought if I could get him to explain his statement, I would have something to grab onto so I could create my rebuttal. No matter how much I pressed him, he just repeated, "That doesn't work for me." I did not get my way.

I got to thinking about it. The phrase had no judgment in it; it was just a perfect stop sign. And I noticed he never said, "I'm sorry, that doesn't work for me." He had no apology for setting a boundary. I stored all this information with the intent to try it out if the opportunity came.

And it did. A few days later, my boss came to me with a nutty idea that would mean a lot of labor and time for me, and I said, with my heart in my throat, "That doesn't work for me." My boss just shrugged and said, "Okay, we'll do something else." He walked away, leaving me amazed at how well that had worked.

Setting boundaries was something I didn't do much as a nicotine user. It was easier to walk away and smoke than to deal with an issue. But I have learned new ways of taking care of myself as a result of Nicotine Anonymous' Steps and Tools. The program has taught me how to set healthy boundaries.

Today, I will set boundaries without judgment
and change the things I can.

SEPTEMBER 27

I was in a tug-of-war between control and letting go.
—Nicotine Anonymous Member

I believed nicotine provided a means of control rather than causing my life to be out of control. In those early months of letting go of nicotine, I felt so out of control when I was stressed and pressed to respond to my life situations. Well-wired thoughts in my head told me, "Inhale nicotine and you'll be able to control everything within a seven second rush."

It was like a tug-of-war that tore me apart. Denial kept me from the truth that nicotine controlled me. I called another NicA member to talk about it, and it became apparent what I was experiencing was straight up fear. One reaction to fear is to freeze and not act. Being in a tug-of-war, I was frozen, stuck.

I needed to act. What to do? I read in "The Serenity Prayer for Nicotine Users" pamphlet, "Remember, it is not really the stress, frustration or even the craving that causes us to keep using nicotine again, but rather our lack of serenity and courage to deal with the craving." Aha, I needed to use the program's solutions and not let the nicotine problem use me. That's letting go, with control.

Today, I focus on the next right thing to do.

SEPTEMBER 28

I choose love because hate is too big a burden to carry.
—Martin Luther King, Jr.

My addictions cost me many relationships. I was a very nasty person when I was on nicotine. I remember being very angry and letting anger fuel my energy. I lost some valuable relationships because I could not contain my anger with myself or others. I blamed everyone and everything else; they caused my anger and fueled my resentments. My denial was so strong that I could not see my part in it. I was choosing this craziness!

I got a quit going for a while, got upset, relapsed, but nicotine didn't numb my emotions. In fact, it did nothing for me. I hated how I felt and had no clue how to deal with life on life's terms without nicotine.

They said to **Keep Showing Up** at meetings even if you are still using, because Nicotine Anonymous will ruin your enjoyment of using nicotine. Gratefully, that has been true for me.

Actively participating in my own recovery has changed me into a more loving and kinder person. I started making some appropriate apologies. I have healthier relationships and pay attention to my part of issues that arise. I actually love, appreciate, and accept myself for the first time. It's been a couple of years now, and I just love being nicotine-free.

Today, I feel, give, and receive the love so freely given to me.

SEPTEMBER 29

Nicotine abuse is insidious,
and slowly eats away at your confidence and self-esteem.
—Nicotine Anonymous Member

I wanted to quit smoking for a long time and sometimes I would even say, "I hate that I smoke!" However, I have memories of moments when I said, "I love to smoke," and my favorite times, like after a meal or maybe before going to sleep. I'm aware I still have the romance lingering long after the parting.

Addiction to nicotine is like being in an emotionally abusive relationship in which no matter how poorly someone is treating me, I feel I need them more. How many times did I keep lighting them up? There was no satisfaction, no pleasure, but I kept chasing after it. I struggled and hoped that if given another chance, the next one might be better, or at least enough to justify going through all the abuse.

Newcomers keep the struggle fresh in my mind. They remind me of the beginning when I wanted to start repairing my life, but didn't have NicA's Tools, a plan, or a clue how to step out of the abuse. Meetings work, in part, because we all have our individual perspective to share and witness, as well as a bond in our common purpose, to be free of nicotine.

Today, I have the wisdom to know the difference between self-care and self-abuse.

We are learning to swim, rather than trying to hold back the tide.
—Nicotine Anonymous Member

Before joining Nicotine Anonymous, I often resisted and fought things I could not change. Accepting life on life's terms was a whole new idea. It took this addiction and my failed attempts at freedom to finally surrender. Thankfully, I found members' support as I surrendered to a Higher Power. I had a safety net and a plan to recover—if only I would become willing to give it a chance.

Life's truths are a tidal force. Instead of swimming against that force, I accepted the sanity of being honest, open, and willing to flow with the tide. Letting go of nicotine and the lies that had poisoned my mind had terrified me for years. Now, I have a fellowship to use as my boat and a spiritual power that moves me forward.

I continue to learn how to surrender, but the serenity and improvements it provides keep showing me its value and purpose. The Serenity Prayer is short and easy to remember, yet powerful. It provides the wisdom to navigate my recovery journey, one day at a time.

Today, I accept the truths that direct me to amend my ways, and provide a healing for myself and others.

OCTOBER 1

Continued to take personal inventory
and when we were wrong promptly admitted it.
— Step Ten

When I first started using nicotine, I saw it as a means to show off my ability to do what I wanted and impress others. Nicotine accented my reactivity and attitudes as I blew smoke at life. However, over time, it just wasn't working for me anymore.

Nicotine addiction injured more than my body; it also injured my relationships. Each time I used nicotine, my attitude toward myself and others was affected. My inability to stop using nicotine continually reminded me of what I couldn't do.

Now, as I work the Steps, I feel encouraged about my ability to create good experiences in my daily life. When I practice this program's principles, I have healthier attitudes and behavior. My saner actions produce better results and show my ability to develop better relationships. I've become more comfortable with who I see in the mirror. Using a daily Tenth Step, I continue to take my personal inventory, admitting when I do wrong, acknowledging when I do right. I respond to life events with more clarity and mindfulness. I like having this kind of integrity.

Today, my healthier attitudes lift me
to new abilities and a new sense of self.

OCTOBER 2

The problem is not the situation,
but how one handles the situation.
—Pir Vilayat Inayat Khan

Situations are not the problem. Living, by its nature, is a series of situations which is a reality I cannot change. But I can effectively influence my life's experience in my attitude and behavior toward these situations. I can either battle life's situations, or accept them as opportunities to expand my talents and practice the program's principles in all my affairs.

Each day I practice being accountable by doing a Tenth Step. I am aided by the clarity of my Fourth Step inventory that revealed what works and what doesn't work. My challenge is to maintain my focus on working the solution, rather than on what I see as a problem.

Using the Serenity Prayer as a guide, I can apply my efforts to what will have a positive effect. This is how I cooperate with my Higher Power in being restored to sanity. I find success in following the spiritual solution of the Serenity Prayer to help me handle most any situation.

Today, success comes from accepting life's situations and shifting my attitude to a spiritual solution.

OCTOBER 3

Disagreement shakes us out of our slumbers
and forces us to see our own point of view through
contrast with another person who does not share it.
—R.D. Laing

Disagreements with others were a trigger situation for me to use nicotine. Disagreements meant I was in direct contact with another in conflict, and I needed a defensive shield and an offensive weapon. Disagreements could also prod me into self-examination that was often uncomfortable. Nicotine was my comforting companion.

My smoke-filled rooms kept me from seeing the truth. When I was confronted with life's challenges without the benefit of having sought a conscious relationship with a Higher Power, I reached instead for the pack in my shirt pocket, conveniently placed over my heart. I even believed I loved them, but today no more.

Now, meetings are a place to practice letting my defenses down. Without fear of criticism, I can take a fresh look at how I conduct myself. When I act poorly, I catch myself and admit I was wrong. When I have differences with others, I act in a more respectful, open minded way. I can better accept that another person can also have a valid point of view.

Today, even if I don't agree, I accept others' views,
and find no reason to use nicotine.

OCTOBER 4

Emotional maturity means not making excuses for yourself.
It means taking responsibility, and avoiding the shortcuts in life.
—John P. Weiss

While I was smoking, I was reactive and would light up at the slightest change in my emotions. Up and down, up and down, as though my feelings were a roller coaster and I was a smokestack. I pointed the finger and blamed everyone else, in total denial of my responsibility for my own behavior. I had no relationship with a Power greater than me.

By the time I found NicA, I was desperate, hurting, spiritually bankrupt, and emotionally exhausted from the struggle. I wanted what these people in recovery had: freedom, joy, serenity! They were laughing and actually enjoying life, nicotine free.

As I quit and the toxins left my body, my pent-up emotions did too. My sponsor and fellow members reminded me that if I'm feeling, I'm healing. I began to feel and accept the feelings instead of stuffing and numbing them with nicotine.

I learned to surrender my reactivity to my Higher Power and take responsibility for my actions. Taking a Tenth Step daily moves me to focus on my part, make amends, and stand tall in my growing emotional maturity.

Today, I take care of my side of the street,
and allow others to take care of theirs.

OCTOBER 5

Settle one difficulty, and you keep a hundred others away.
—Chinese Proverb

Although the fellowship's primary purpose is to support each other's quest to be free of nicotine, we also want to live with more joy. I know that requires more than just not putting nicotine in my body. It is important to work the Steps to see how my shortcomings and my difficulties are connected.

I've experienced making progress with one shortcoming involving a resentment. I responded differently to one situation, and I saw how a chain reaction of improvement rippled through my life. By letting go of an old resentment, I removed something that previously had me act judgmental and critical. This change helped me to see other shortcomings I had overlooked before.

Doing my Step Ten inventory each day reveals how my difficulties can snowball if I don't address a shortcoming. I know I have work to do, and I have a program and sponsor to help me. I work at my own pace daily. I keep making the effort, and I trust many more good results will come.

Today, I build awareness about my shortcomings,
and when appropriate work a Tenth Step.

OCTOBER 6

We need to maintain constant vigilance
so we don't reactivate our addiction.
—Nicotine Anonymous "Slogans" pamphlet

"Our Promises" remind us that "We begin to forget we had been nicotine users, except at meetings." I enjoy being free of nicotine, but I should not forget my addiction so that I don't slip back into it.

Forgetting is a recurring problem for me. Fairly new at this program, I'm in the early stages of abstaining from nicotine. When a craving strikes, I can forget I have NicA's Tools to use instead of using nicotine. My mind goes blank, except for obsessing about my source of nicotine. I want to remember I have NicA alternatives.

I've started to put up sticky notes at different locations in my home, my car, and my job site. I've written excerpts from our Steps and Traditions, literature, NicA's five Tools, the Serenity Prayer, and the Third Step Prayer. My memos include slogans such as **Look for the Lesson**, and **Lengths Become Strengths**. I tape my group's phone/email list to my refrigerator. From the NicA "Tips for Gaining Freedom" pamphlet, I learned that it helps if I pray instead of puff and take a second look before I react. With practice, I begin to trust that I will keep remembering to use the Tools of recovery that helped me gain freedom from nicotine.

Today, I remember I was addicted to nicotine
so I do not forget to go to my meeting.

OCTOBER 7

I wish I had known that I could stop smoking one day for
one moment at a time, because I thought I had to smoke.

—Nicotine Anonymous Member

I believed I did not have any choice but to smoke. I tried to stop so many times and failed each time. Being in another 12-Step program did not help. I would pray and pray and still continue to smoke.

One day, I was heading to a meeting and instead drove to the hospital, because I couldn't breathe. My body shut down and I ended up in intensive care for two weeks. Here again, my freedom of choice was taken away from me.

I got out of the hospital and started applying the Twelve Steps this time for nicotine as I used them for alcohol. After nine months of being nicotine free, I started going to Nicotine Anonymous meetings, because I was going crazy and wanted nicotine.

I attended meetings regularly, got a sponsor, worked the Steps of Nicotine Anonymous, and started helping others. I have not had to use nicotine since then.

Today, I have a choice I did not have
until I came to Nicotine Anonymous.

OCTOBER 8

When I think of others who are suffering more than I am,
I become more compassionate and understanding.
I approach others with kindness.
—Nicotine Anonymous Member

My sponsor recently made me aware of this principle after I complained about how long it was taking for an application for services to be processed. She mentioned the fact that the workers are probably overwhelmed with paperwork. My complaint was self-centered. I overcame my bad attitude by focusing on their situation and finding compassion.

I appreciate being treated with kindness and benefit from being nurturing and kind to myself. Taking care of myself, I am better able to help others. I make healthy food choices, exercise, drink water, and deep breathe.

When I am in pain, I go to any length to avoid using nicotine again, because this too shall pass. My miracle is happening, in my Higher Power's time, not mine.

I am no longer alone. I offer to help others in a kindly manner. I reach out via phone, email, instant message, and text. When I offer kindness to others, the gift of reaching out is that I am relieved of the bondage of self.

Today, I reach out and am kind to others.
I am also good to myself.

OCTOBER 9

I need to pause and not act out on my triggered emotions.
—Nicotine Anonymous Member

When I get pissed off, I get defensive and/or I withdraw. From this, I build a barricade of resentment, mindlessly accepting my behavior as a solution. It never was a solution. What went unresolved turned the anger inward towards myself with feelings of my own incompetence. I reached for my poison of choice to numb my emotions as the ultimate solution. Now, I see this is insanity. I have admitted so many ways that nicotine made my life unmanageable.

I am humbled. Slowly but surely, I am accepting that what I had "proudly viewed as self-reliance was really arrogance, rebelliousness, defiance, and denial." Rather than letting emotions get all pent up, I let go and let Good Orderly Direction guide my responses. It's wiser to discuss than to do damage. Doing so lessens the amends I have to make each day.

Now, instead of taking a deep inhale of nicotine, I can pause by taking a deep breath. After all, how many of my "smoke breaks" were pauses I needed? Now, I call my sponsor. We say the Serenity Prayer and seek wisdom that makes a difference. Together, we pause to make conscious contact with our Higher Power of our own understanding. That provides spiritual order to an emotional disorder, and life becomes manageable.

Today, I pause and ask for the serenity, courage, and wisdom that helps make my life more manageable.

OCTOBER 10

You bring about what you think about.
And so, if you can control what you think about,
all else will fall into place—
friends, laughter, prosperity, fulfillment, and love.
—Mike Dooley

If I can control what I think about, that means I have a choice. So, if I don't like the thought I'm thinking, I can choose a better thought.t

Addiction to nicotine controlled my thoughts for several decades. It seemed like I had no control over my thoughts. My continual thought was when I would get my next fix, did I have enough cigarettes to last until tomorrow, or where is my lighter? Nicotine was my higher power and I had few thoughts that weren't born of that incessant urge to use nicotine.

"Our Promises" do come true, despite the fact that the addiction still lurks. My only thoughts of using nicotine occur when I'm at meetings. I need to remember I am an addict and always will be. I am learning to pay attention to my thoughts. Better thoughts lead to better behavior. Clearly, my life is better now that I am accountable for my behavior.

I want to share life's pleasures with others: friends, laughter, prosperity, fulfillment, and love. That's what living is now all about.

---

*Today, I think happy thoughts,
act responsibly, and attract goodness into my life.*

OCTOBER 11

Strength can come from acknowledging our resistance
and may provide us with the humility
that may be necessary in asking for help.
—Nicotine Anonymous: The Book

Before I quit, I practiced my version of the 5 Ds (Delay, Distract, Discuss, Drink water, Deep breathe) for several weeks just to see what it would be like to respond differently to a craving. I asked my Higher Power for the serenity to wait until a craving subsided. Each time I was able to delay using nicotine a little more.

After several weeks of attending meetings, reading the literature, working the Steps with my sponsor, doing service work, and practicing the 5 Ds, I finally set a quit date. It was scary, because I couldn't imagine coping without nicotine. Running to nicotine was how I reacted to life.

Acknowledging my resistance, I was encouraged to be proactive, so I planned out the quit day. I wanted to be distracted and be where I could not use nicotine. That plan fell through, I found a nicotine device, and used it. Still, with my NicA group cheering me on with **Keep Showing Up**. They assured me that with willingness to be willing, I would get my miracle. I did.

Practicing paid off for me, because once I quit, I was well prepared. I felt assured having my Higher Power, the group, the Tools, and my sponsor to support me when life got stressful. It's working because I work it.

---

*Today, I have the courage to be proactive
and to use the Tools of the program to live nicotine free.*

OCTOBER 12

Despite everything, I believe that people are really good at heart.
—Anne Frank

As I have learned to accept my own mistakes and allow myself to be human, I have also begun to develop compassion for myself and for others. I can see that most other people are actually doing the best they can to get through this world, just the way I am. If they have a program, I also know they are working on themselves and are likely to make their own amends in their own time. If they are not working a program, I can actually view them with compassion, remembering how life was for me before I came to NicA.

The beautiful process of making amends has taught me both forgiveness and compassion not only for other people, but for myself as well. As I clean up my life, I mature emotionally and realize that all those old ideas I had about how all of us needed to be were just that: ideas of mine, and not necessarily facts.

Of course, I am still nowhere near perfect and don't expect to get there in this lifetime. As I continue taking a daily inventory, I see progress with more easily overcoming my character flaws. I continue to stay honest about my defects and ask for help in making the necessary adjustments as I go.

Today, I work to keep my side of the street clean
and strive to have compassion for myself and those around me.

OCTOBER 13

I do not at all understand the mystery of grace,
only that it meets us where we are
but does not leave us where it found us.
—Anne Lamott

It took me twenty years after my first hit of nicotine to stop using it. I quit when, mysteriously, I stopped feeling cravings. I had never thought of myself as a nicotine addict in those years, because on many days I didn't use it. I paid no attention to other days when I used more nicotine than usual.

Years after my last hit of nicotine, I became involved with another 12-Step program, which encouraged me to revisit my nicotine history. I became acquainted with Nicotine Anonymous, read its literature, and learned that I have an addiction. I learned about people who relapsed after years of not using, and that I am at risk of going back to using nicotine again. I learned the fellowship accepts people who have quit but are worried about relapse.

I read the Steps aloud during my first meeting. When I introduced myself and heard my own voice say, "I am powerless over nicotine," I finally got it. I finally understood how the grace of my Higher Power moved me to stop using nicotine years before, right where I was.

Today, I meet myself in recovery and find
the mystery of grace in my Higher Power.

OCTOBER 14

I expected things to change without changing anything I did,
and without even knowing what, or how, to change.
Nicotine Anonymous Member

I was a fairly rational person capable of solving everyday problems. However, when it came to my nicotine addiction, I was a confused coward stuck in the muck of denial and at risk of becoming one of the millions of nicotine-related deaths each year. I wanted to quit nicotine, but my addicted brain wanted more nicotine. My willpower screamed, "I will have nicotine!" Left on my own, I was clueless and unwilling to change, nor to go where I had not gone before.

Recovery has been a process. First, I admitted that on my own, I was powerless over nicotine. Next, I came to believe I would recover by turning over my willfulness in exchange for the guidance of a Power greater than myself. Then, it came time to take a daring look in the mirror and write an inventory of my strengths and my weaknesses. I revealed them all to my sponsor, especially those insecurities that kept me hidden behind a nicotine screen. I assessed those character traits and decided whether to keep or discard them. This process has given me confidence that with spiritual guidance and this fellowship of support, I can learn to change myself, the only thing I can change, and hold myself accountable one day at a time.

Today, guided by the wisdom I've gained, I continue to change,
and find the peace I have always sought.

OCTOBER 15

Friendship with oneself is all important,
because without it one cannot be friends
with anyone else in the world.
—Eleanor Roosevelt

When I battled ol' nicodemon early in my quit, I made a list of all the things I could do besides smoke. Was I ever surprised that the list was so easy to write! There were so many other wonderful things to do that were soothing, healthy, and even healing.

I love the water, so one mild afternoon, I took my dog to the river. We walked along the water, played fetch, and enjoyed quiet time under the towering sycamores. I drew in my sketchbooks and wrote letters to my Higher Power.

I realized I could have anything in the entire universe except nicotine. It felt like the floodgates of life were opening wide, and all I had to do was jump into the flow.

It took courage and time. As I worked the Steps, the smokescreen lifted, enabling me to focus on being my own friend. Now, I can also be a friend to members of a worldwide fellowship called Nicotine Anonymous.

Today, I take moments of self-care and reflect
on improving the friendship with myself and others.

OCTOBER 16

"I think, therefore I am," is the statement of an intellectual
who underrates toothaches.
"I feel, therefore I am," is a truth much more universally valid,
and it applies to everything that's alive.
—Milan Kundera

I tried to think my way out of addiction. I used nicotine whenever I had a negative thought. When lonely, I'd reach for my friend nicotine. When angry with someone, I would use nicotine to spite them. Convinced my troubles went away when I used nicotine, I repeatedly drugged my thoughts and feelings with nicotine for years. This clouded my perception of what was real, and what was my distortion. That, I've learned, was part of nicotine's addictive trap.

I had let my stinking thinking deceive me into acting self- destructively. This made me feel weak, dispirited, and hopeless. The real cause of the problem was my disrespect and dishonesty with myself and the people around me.

As I began to serve others and to humbly and honestly perform loving, forgiving, accepting, and spiritual acts, the trap that nicotine set for me was shattered. The way out was simply to stop thinking about it, and to get busy, act as if, and do what a nicotine-free person does.

Today, I am grateful for the clarity gained about my addiction, and the opportunity to make amends to myself and others.

OCTOBER 17

I need to refrain from crosstalk in my own mind.
—Nicotine Anonymous Member

How I was in the past kept chattering in my inner ear. I found it difficult to be the recovering person I am now in each present moment. Although it's essential to work at my shortcomings, I also needed to own the progress I've made as a result of working the Twelve Steps. It was time to update my personal résumé and to embrace a new perspective of the healing, recovering, spiritual being I was becoming.

As I'm learning to manage my memories—the good, the bad, and the ugly—I may still have a memory that feels like a craving for nicotine. It wants to nudge me to act out one of my shortcomings. A powerful memory may create an urgency that presses at me to respond the way I had before.

But now, I'm committed, that my response is that I no longer use nicotine. I'm also practicing more positive responses to the daily challenges of living. I no longer accept my former excuses as reasons to use. Those excuses just led to the same old patterns that I've admitted are not rational and no longer work for me. I'm in the business of creating new memories that speak to me of who I have become in the present. That's a gift.

Today, right this moment, I am free to change who I am and how I am doing.

OCTOBER 18

Would you like to feel better?
Then reach for a better feeling or thought.
—Louise Hay

Before and during my early recovery, my focus was reacting to what was going on around me. I was incredibly sensitive. I focused on what others were doing instead of what was going on within me and my own responsibilities.

I took action and worked the Steps with my sponsor, did service work, read literature, and reached out to others. Gradually, I was able to focus my attention on my own recovery and not what everyone else was doing.

I have no idea what someone else is going through. And really, where do I want to put my energy? If my priority is my own recovery, my job is to keep my focus on my responsibilities. My thinking and actions are the only thing I have any control over. My job is to improve the habits of my mind and my own behavior.

With practice, I'm learning to take actions that improve my mental and emotional wellbeing, and I feel better. My spiritual life is not a theory, I live it.

Today, I reach for the Tools of the program
to feel better and behave better toward myself and others.

OCTOBER 19

You are a child of the universe
no less than the trees and the stars;
you have a right to be here.
—The Desiderata

I can feel good about myself just because I exist. That's it. I don't have to make excuses or justify. I am lovable, I deserve love. Loving my sweet soul is the best way to express my Higher Power's love for me, and for me to be able to love others.

Comparing myself to others brings up old, tired messages that I'm not good enough. That's not the truth. I am good enough, and so is everyone else.

Now in recovery, I am no longer afraid that I won't be accepted, or that I'll end up alone and forsaken. Members of my group have loved me into loving myself. I have been shown how it's possible to be in acceptance and appreciation for what is, right this moment, right here right now, and not worry about the rest.

Today, all I have to do is put down the nicotine,
and I receive the many gifts of recovery.
I am one blessed soul.

OCTOBER 20

Slips start in my head, well before I light up.
If I don't deal with it, it's just a matter of time.
—Nicotine Anonymous Member

I was used to drifting off from reality on trails of smoke and living in my head. I believed I could handle anything with a little mental juggling. Nicotine enabled me to ignore and numb my feelings. When life pushed, I pulled back into my head to isolate myself. I backed myself into corners with nothing to reach out for but my drug.

Isolation puts my recovery in jeopardy. Isolation has no witnesses and risks thinking, "It doesn't matter, nobody will know." Eventually, alone and deprived, I'll feel justified to have at least one.

Now in recovery, I guard against such thoughts and situations. I stay focused on the truth because once I light one, I ignite both my mental obsession and nicotine's power to suck me into the endless cycle of addiction.

Nicotine addiction is a disease of the body, mind, and spirit. If I let my mind begin to wander from the program's principles or to romance the notion that, "I could have just one," I am beginning a nosedive back into the agonizing pit of addiction. And so, I pay attention to the alarm bells and allow the program's saving grace to help me keep my mind focused on the next right thing.

Today, I commit to not pick up what will make me fall down.

OCTOBER 21

Each group has but one primary purpose—
to carry its message to the nicotine addict who still suffers.
—Tradition Five

I knew I wanted to stop smoking. I hated spending money for my fix. Still, I thought I was in control and had a choice when to light up to relax. I was wrong. It was the addiction that was calling the shots. I was merely surrendering my will to an insidious master and contributing to its corporate coffers through my daily consumption of its product, no matter how high the price.

I found relief from this bondage in Nicotine Anonymous meetings. I felt welcome. These people understood what I was facing, supported me to get my quit going, and told me to **Keep Showing Up**. No matter how rough the cravings got, my friends in NicA helped me through them.

At a NicA meeting soon after my last hit of nicotine, I felt elated when I noticed I barely had any nicotine stains on my fingers. It was a physical sign that I was beginning to recover from my former master's bondage.

I didn't understand what a gift freedom was until I received it. At one time, I could only go a few hours without thinking about using nicotine. Soon, the time between those thoughts became months. I no longer needed to leave my friends to go outside and feed my addiction. I have been freed of the obsession, and gratefully accept the gifts of recovery.

Today, I respect my quit and what a gift it is to be free.

OCTOBER 22

The map of life can change in a split second,
we just have to deal with the road we choose.
—Nicotine Anonymous Member

Thanks to Nicotine Anonymous I now know that nicotine and I could never be besties again. When I was using, I kept believing the lie that nicotine solved problems, and I wouldn't have to feel the pain.

I thought my life and my entire world had exploded twice in one month, because two of the people who are very dear to me died from cancer. These two were my family, my life. I had been chain smoking a pack and a half every day for 31 years, and those losses changed my ability to cope. I upped the ante and started smoking so much that my own health problems began. This changed my life. I had to choose between hurting myself or changing my life to get free of nicotine.

I am now living my new normal, without nicotine. In part, it's an amends to my dearly departed. My sponsor tells me I'm now **Dealing with the Feeling**. Our "Slogans" pamphlet reminds me: "Recovery also provides us with the opportunity to feel new joys." I am dealing with feelings, uncomfortable and wonderful. This is what it's like to be a spiritual being having a human experience, and each day I'm a better human for it.

Today, I choose this beautiful new nicotine-free world,
and fully feel my humanness.

OCTOBER 23

You gain strength, courage, and confidence by every experience
in which you really stop to look fear in the face.

—Eleanor Roosevelt

We try...

by staying in today,
by staying nicotine free for today,
one day, one moment, one breath
at a time, and by letting our Higher Power in

We try...

by loving ourselves and our neighbors,
by getting out of self with compassion,
by setting boundaries with the people we love

We try...

by living in the now,
by living in the breath of life,
by volunteering our love

We try...

by putting aside the fear, by jumping in that cold water and finding it wasn't so bad after all, by standing tall, breathing deeply and knowing it's going to be okay.

---

*Today, I have the courage to live outside of my comfort zone,
love myself, do what I never thought possible.
I ask for help and I am free.*

OCTOBER 24

I was proud to be a "hard core" smoker. How foolish.

—Nicotine Anonymous: The Book

When I began to review my pre-recovery "movie," I saw much foolishness. Years of deluding myself about my smoking filled my daily script with excuses and rationalizations. The repetitive scenes of deceiving myself, much less others, got written up in my Fourth Step inventory. I admitted how my actions were wrong and often hurtful. At first, there was only shame attached to my past.

Making living amends in my daily life now gives me a chance to change. Lessons learned and practiced have become guiding wisdom. As I attend Nicotine Anonymous meetings, I learn that my experience as a nicotine addict enables me to have deeper compassion for myself and my fellow members. I learn the sense of mutual identification and connection is how much of our learning happens in relationships.

My addiction, along with my desire to gain freedom, brought me to NicA. Its program and members are the best school I've ever attended. Thankfully, because I had been such a fool, I have gained much wisdom. Service opportunities in NicA and my community allow me to give back wisdom I've gathered. It's a transformative experience having a better director on my set.

Today, I continually gain wisdom from my foolishness.

Addiction once had me automatically reaching
for another hit of nicotine;
now I automatically reach for a NicA Tool.
—Nicotine Anonymous Member

I first heard, "We seek progress not perfection" at Nicotine Anonymous meetings. In hindsight, my first tiny bit of progress was reaching the meeting, though I was still smoking before and after. The next bit was reaching out to accept the service of opening the door to the meeting, though I was still smoking. Eventually, I began to reach for the NicA literature and the phone list to call members between meetings, still smoking. At the time, I didn't really appreciate any of that as progress because I hadn't achieved my goal to stop smoking.

I continued on automatic pilot, reaching for a cigarette, still stuck in the same flight pattern. However, I was becoming much more conscious of my behavior and my true desire to land in that promised land where we begin to forget we had been nicotine users, except at meetings.

That continuing commitment enabled me to reach nicotine freedom. Now, I automatically reach for NicA Tools as part of my daily personal inventory and spiritual maintenance. I focus on NicA rather than nicotine. I remain humbly grateful for this gift of freedom from nicotine.

Today, I consciously continue to seek progress in my life.

OCTOBER 26

Without willing members, I have no meeting
for support or to hold myself accountable.
—Nicotine Anonymous Member

Members' attendance at meetings fulfills several purposes for me. Members' presence each week sustains the group's existence. That bolsters my faith that there will be a meeting next week. How would I ever keep learning without hearing the deep and authentic shares of my fellow members' voices? I would not have the connection with a Power greater than myself without my members' inspiration and support, or their adherence to the principle that my spirituality is of my own understanding.

I also need members to be my witnesses. I'm early into this recovery process, still on a trial basis. I don't know yet if I can trust my own perceptions of myself. I still need others to validate when I do right, because I tend to think I haven't done enough or I've gone overboard. I'm still fumbling forward with the Steps, yet committed to sharing my truth. Members' presence helps to hold me accountable for my thoughts and actions, and whether or not I am headed toward a relapse. I need a check system to keep me balanced. Members are my gentle jury of my peers who hear me out. My Higher Power sentences me to a lifetime of support.

Today, I'm grateful I can get a witness. Amen!

OCTOBER 27

We are either working on recovery
or we are working on a relapse.
—Nicotine Anonymous Member

Before attending NicA meetings, I didn't realize that so many of my negative behaviors and feelings were actually due to unconscious choices I made. By continually repeating them, they became habitual, much like addiction. I wasn't using my consciousness. No wonder my life was unmanageable, I wasn't managing my life; my habitual behavior was managing me.

I came to accept cravings for nicotine, and I changed how I responded. Clearly, if I didn't choose to change my response to the cravings, I would fall back into my addiction.

Recovery has brought me to my senses. I became more conscious that I had choices in how I respond to my experiences, as well as make choices for how I initiate my experiences. When I feel deprived, I refocus and connect with what I already have. I can also start my day reciting my gratitude list.

My sponsor shared how conscious practice eventually becomes habit forming. The more I practice, the more readily I'll choose a response or create an initiative to have a better experience for myself. To gain the full benefits of recovery requires my willing efforts and active consciousness.

---

*Today, I make conscious choices to improve
and maintain my recovery.*

OCTOBER 28

When I was using nicotine, I was bitter and nothing mattered.
Now everything matters.
—Nicotine Anonymous Member

During my initial time of letting go of nicotine, I discovered I could actually get angry. I became less likely to react my usual way to disturbances with, "Oh, that's okay, I don't mind, it doesn't matter" to avoid conflict. Part of me knew those denied feelings would drain into an inner resentment reservoir and breed bitterness. This often led to passive aggressive behaviors or depression resulting in even more unmanageability in relationships.

Nicotine certainly maintained a bitter taste in my mouth. However, did my mouth speak with bitter words? Did I have a hidden bitter character trait exposed in my personal inventory?

Working the Steps put me in conscious contact with a part of me that knows the truth about many things I do and their consequences. Yet, as with the insanity of addiction, I kept reacting the same way, expecting and wishing for different results.

Following the guidance of this program, along with therapy, I've been practicing and learning skills to better respond to conflicts. I seek humble solutions rather than victories by subterfuge. Change has been a matter of willingness and courage.

Today, to taste the sweetness of being happy, joyous, and free.
I accept that everything I do matters.

OCTOBER 29

There was no way to hide, and the very attempt was a lie.
—Nicotine Anonymous: The Book

After I stopped smoking, I felt as though I had taken off my clothes. During those first days and weeks of the big change, it was as if I was stark naked trying to cope with my life without nicotine. I felt exposed and vulnerable. The unmasking was so uncomfortable and confusing, yet it felt so real. I realized how much I had used nicotine to cover up my insecurities and deaden my emotions.

And I couldn't hide the fact I was addicted to nicotine, and without nicotine, it felt as if I had lost my cover. I had to learn to dress with a new wardrobe that fit who I really am, warts and all. That took time and patience. Without using nicotine, I had more time, but I still had an addict's lack of patience. Developing patience took the help and care of my sponsor and my Higher Power.

"Our Promises" affirm that I was learning to assert myself where previously I have been aggressive or passive. With the courage I ask for, I move forward, **Dealing with the Feelings**.

Today, I welcome my new wardrobe,
and I wear it with integrity.

OCTOBER 30

Thus, we need the serenity to accept the craving,
the courage to just let it pass,
and the wisdom to know the difference.
—*"The Serenity Prayer for Nicotine Users"* pamphlet

My mind plays tricks, not telling me what I need, only what I want. Another form of my insanity is being out of control with unmanageable thoughts. In my initial stages of abstinence, my brain ran rampant, confusing want with need. When my brain thought, "I need nicotine," it was incapable of realizing it was a cunning lie unless I challenged it. It felt like an invisible force was pushing me to go to my local nicotine dealer, as if my very life depended on it. How insane!

I realized I needed to be restored to sanity. Reading the pamphlet, I accepted and recognized "the craving for what it was: a strong desire, physical as psychological, not a real need, for nicotine."

The more I make conscious contact with my thoughts, I realize there are many other situations when I confuse want and need. Clearly, this confusion is a pervasive symptom of my addiction, this disease. This program provides me with a process to fulfill my actual needs and ease my mind and heart.

Today, my life and joy depend on the wisdom
I'm willing to accept.

OCTOBER 31

Go as far as you can see; when you get there,
you'll be able to see further.
—Thomas Carlyle

Before I joined Nicotine Anonymous, I couldn't see past my own smokescreen, both figuratively, and often literally. Despite a deep longing to stop, I couldn't imagine living without nicotine. Self-pity was my familiar comfort zone and how I wallowed in my painful shame.

When I joined NicA, I didn't have a clue of what was ahead or how I would ever get there, wherever *there* was. I listened to members' experience, strength, and hope. I came to realize it was normal to be unable to imagine not using nicotine. I had smoked for many years and had been exposed to my parents' secondhand smoke since conception. Nicotine had even stunted my imagination!

When I heard, "We need to become willing to go to any length," I made a decision to show up at meetings no matter what. At first, that was as far as I could see. Gradually I began to suspect the possibility that I could live without nicotine. With the care I got from members at each meeting, I increasingly saw freedom more clearly. I finally gained my freedom beyond what I could ever have imagined.

Today, I will have faith there is more goodness ahead than I can see from here.

NOVEMBER 1

If I practice the meditation part of Step Eleven,
I will understand what my Higher Power has to offer.
—Nicotine Anonymous Member

When I was smoking, I was fussing and fuming. The chemicals pushed me up or held me down. I couldn't see the forest through the smog. There was no patience in this craving person. I only looked busy, I was not really achieving the peace and understanding that I truly wanted.

When I practice the meditation part of Step Eleven, I understand what my Higher Power has to offer. It is only in this deep silence that I can hear the deep messages.

Working the Steps leading up to the Eleventh Step helps me clear away the noises that can clutter up my honesty, openness, and willingness. As I let go, stay still and wait, the many gifts of serenity alight. I practice conscious contact with my HP, and my life flows. I achieve the peace and understanding I truly want.

Today, I welcome the quiet and receive the gifts of serenity, peace, and understanding from my Higher Power.

NOVEMBER 2

In every walk with nature
one receives far more than he seeks.
—John Muir

No longer chained to nicotine, I love walking outside and observing plants and animals in nature. My attitude improves, I feel closer to my Higher Power, and I return to being filled with the wonder of creation. I believe my HP expresses the abundance and beauty of creation through nature.

I breathe in the freshness of the air and the sweet aromas of plants and trees—they are gifts of recovery. I see a sparkle of sunlight off water, trace the beautiful patterns in leaves and touch the soft mosses, while the birdsong rises in chorus. Everywhere life is growing, moving, and so fully alive.

When walking with my Higher Power in nature, I often sort through my thoughts and feelings, and listen for HP's will. I return to my work refreshed, assured of the good that's happening in my life.

Today, I make time to seek my Higher Power in nature.

NOVEMBER 3

A spiritual path is about asking questions,
not seeking certainty through answers.
—Sarah Bowen

An essential reason I could become and remain a member of Nicotine Anonymous was the principle that my spiritual beliefs were to be of my own understanding. Neither the fellowship nor any one member would dictate the what and how of my spiritual beliefs.

I enjoy science for whatever certainty it may provide about the wonders all around me. Spirituality is my canvas to paint about those wonders however I am inspired. My spiritual journey is a book with some written chapters, but many blank pages are left for pondering.

I'm comfortable with my beliefs when and as they work for me. They're based on principled purposes. I accept that my beliefs have no claim to absolute certainty. I don't even desire to seek certainty's end. I prefer open wondering rather than closing my beliefs in a box. Experience has shown me what happens in life doesn't always fit into boxes. I question, therefore I am.

Nicotine Anonymous has given me freedom from nicotine and freedom to believe, while in a supportive community of diverse believers who are each equally free.

Today, I am gratefully responsible for the spiritual path of my own understanding.

NOVEMBER 4

So you've quit smoking!
Now what are you going to do with the rest of your life?
—Nicotine Anonymous Member

I tried so hard to outsmart it, but it almost outsmarted me. I thought no one knew I smoked. Well, I hoped no one knew, but sometimes the looks I got confirmed my worst fear. Eventually everyone knew.

Now, I've quit smoking. And I know I didn't do it alone. As I think about this great gift of grace and freedom, I thank those in my fellowship who carried me through the darkness into light.

So much time was lost hiding my addiction. Now, I am brave enough to walk up to someone who patted me on the back with a word of encouragement, or to say hello to the quiet person who didn't say much but placed a phone number into my hand after the meeting.

Tonight, before the starlight fades, I'll offer my sincere gratitude to God for putting Nicotine Anonymous in my life. I whisper, "Thanks, God. I've quit smoking. We did it!"

Today, I will not take my quit for granted,
nor the power of my Nicotine Anonymous group!

NOVEMBER 5

If we concentrate on praying for and performing God's will,
our own petty desires and egotistical wants start to diminish.
We become more serene and flow with our
own essential nature.

—Nicotine Anonymous: The Book

How do I know what my Higher Power's will for me is? How can I focus on that as I move through the various parts of my day? For me, the God of my understanding is benevolent, and I trust in this goodness. This means my HP wants me to feel good, think good thoughts, and spread goodness throughout my day to all I encounter.

I learn it's okay to be human and make mistakes along the way. These lessons are my greatest teachers. The irritating coworker, the crazy boss, the circumstances of life, they are all my teachers, and I'm in a learning process called recovery.

Life is a process, and we are going through this together, so each of us chooses how we will respond to what's happening around us. I can choose acceptance of or resistance to life on life's terms. It's my perspective on a situation that paints my response and affects my serenity. I maintain the safe and peaceful place within my heart, my own essential nature, through conscious contact with my Higher Power and by listening carefully.

Today, I do the next right thing, which if I listen carefully,
I trust to be my Higher Power's will for me.

NOVEMBER 6

Lots of folks confuse bad management with destiny.
—Kin Hubbard

I felt like an unpardonable prisoner to my addiction. I used problematic defenses to comfort me. I managed pain and uncomfortable feelings by medicating with my drug. To deny my responsibility, I defended my sense of futility and called it fate. I felt so down on myself that I didn't want to torture myself with the truth.

Then I had a mini stroke. My daughter began to plead with me to try Nicotine Anonymous. I resisted at first, but then relented. I came to realize that my life was unmanageable because it was under bad management, and not that I was destined to fail. Step Three involves turning over the management of my life to the care of a guide, Good Orderly Direction, of my own understanding.

Practicing the Eleventh Step, I seek conscious contact. Through prayer and meditation, I ask for willingness and guidance. In these quiet places I can receive inspiration. Rather than being resigned to fate, I am choosing to have faith in a program that has worked for so many others. If they can manage that, I can.

Today, I am grateful to be under new management.

Spiritual progress comes by changing one's point of view.
—Pir Vilayat Inayat Khan

The cycle of addiction kept bringing me back to a singular point of view, "I must use tobacco." I believed nothing was better than nicotine. I could not allow myself to move beyond its reach. The insanity of this went unchallenged for years.

Recovery has proven that progress requires a willingness to change how I see myself and what I value. I go to meetings to set aside my defenses and let the experience, strength, and hope of others into my heart and mind.

Meetings also give me a safe place to rediscover my own truth. This deeper connection is part of my spiritual experience. As my truth is uncovered, I see myself in a new light, making it easier to change my point of view. The Eleventh Step guides me to have conscious contact with my spiritual source. I have courage to let go and surrender to a deeper level, which increases my spiritual progress.

Today, I move beyond former limits
as new possibilities arise along my spiritual path.

NOVEMBER 8

Swimming is my meditation, one stroke, one breath at a time.
—Nicotine Anonymous Member

I heard a member share how swimming was her way to meditate and create an inner peace. This was a valuable example of the fellowship's openness for each member to come to their own spiritual understanding. I keep listening and learning about other possibilities and ways to make my life more manageable and satisfying without nicotine.

Her regular pool laps led her to twice swim across the Hudson River with a large group of other swimmers. That was inspiring evidence of how recovery manifests a new confidence and an enduring faith to courageously go where one has not gone before. I too have been inspired to go where I had not gone before.

Rather than seek a fixed concept of a spiritual presence, I prefer my own understanding and to remain open to what serves and inspires me in any given moment. I can even borrow from others and let their words lift and support me. I marvel at a meditative moment when I clearly feel a spiritual presence within.

Today, I am open to the spiritual resources in this present moment.

NOVEMBER 9

Be grateful for your life, every detail of it,
and your face will come to shine like a sun...
Persist in gratitude, and you will slowly become
one with the Sun of Love.

—Rumi

When I was using nicotine and trying to quit, I saw myself and everything in my life only in negative terms. I did not like my job, I did not like where I lived, and I was unhappy with my family life.

My unhappiness persisted after I quit. Although I felt relieved that I no longer abused my body and spirit with nicotine, I felt a lot of anger and sadness about my life. After one hysterical email to my sponsor about the latest situation that had upset me, my sponsor suggested I send her a daily gratitude list.

Some time after I started making a daily gratitude list, I had an epiphany. A voice inside me said, "What if you just let yourself enjoy your job?" A cascade of other epiphanies was spiritually delivered. Now I love my life. It is a love born of being grateful for what I have.

I still sometimes struggle with finding something to be grateful for. But I find if I persist, my efforts are always rewarded, and my life continues to open to love.

Today, I focus on what I can be grateful for,
and I shine like a sun.

NOVEMBER 10

When overwhelmed by stress I stop,
turn to my Higher Power and pray and meditate.
I keep letting go and letting God.
—Nicotine Anonymous Member

I will always have stress. It's how I handle it that makes the difference in my serenity and wellbeing. Stress can motivate me at times. I accept it for what it is and move forward on doing the next right thing. Taking this action helps relieve the stress.

I break things down into smaller chunks and do one, then another, one bite at a time. I repeat the Serenity Prayer over and over, and God gives me that extra oomph, right when I need it.

When I get stressed, I shut my thinker off and go into automatic mode and do the next right thing. I accept stress is a part of life. So how am I responding to stress? Am I adding to my own stress? Do I have a bad attitude or get fearful?

Stress drains and strains my body and soul, and smoking will never, ever make it one iota better. Using nicotine will make stress multiply. Stress motivates me or paralyzes me. I get to choose.

Today, God, grant me the serenity
to accept the things I cannot change,
the courage to change the things I can,
and the wisdom to know the difference.

NOVEMBER 11

In my experience, talking with my Higher Power
really helps me turn things over, let go, and grow.
—Nicotine Anonymous Member

I know it's my Higher Power's will for me when I feel serene and peaceful while I am making choices and taking action. Then I can be serene while I let go of the outcome. Often doing this results in the best outcome for all concerned.

Over time, I have learned to differentiate between the feeling of angst when I'm doing my will, and the uncomfortable feeling when I'm behaving in a new healthy way that I'm not used to. I am usually fearful when I'm in my will. Clearly, the discomfort of new healthy behavior is part of growth, like a butterfly bursting forth from its chrysalis. The result is often a beautiful transformation.

When my thoughts begin to spiral out of control, I repeat the Serenity Prayer or the Third Step Prayer, breathe, focus on the meaning of the words of the prayer, and clear my thoughts. I listen to my Higher Power's will for me.

And if I'm really resisting letting go, I call my sponsor, a trusted friend, or member of NicA. My sponsor has helped me see more clearly where I am resisting. I have learned to heed her experience, strength, and hope because I want what she has.

Today, help me listen for my Higher Power's will for me,
and let go of outcomes.

NOVEMBER 12

Heaven means to be one with God.

—Confucius

For me, the purpose of prayer is to get to know God, to be with and communicate with God. It's a reunion with my Higher Power. Through prayer, I link up my soul, mind, and will to God.

When I was learning to pray, I acted as if I knew how. The Third Step and Seventh Step Prayers were helpful when I started out. I made the connection and joined with the God of my understanding, by asking and receiving.

With practice, prayer has become easier for me. I pray at the same time every day, in the morning upon rising and at night upon retiring. I ask for my Higher Power's will for me in morning prayers and thank my Higher Power for all my blessings in evening prayers. It brings me power for daily living and provides me a spiritual reserve. I believe there is no right or wrong way to pray, there is no formula but to make it a habit. When I'm alone, I pray out loud. I see the basis of prayer as, "Thy will be done in me and through me today."

Prayer is one of the many gifts I've received from Nicotine Anonymous. Although I do pray for willingness, serenity, courage, wisdom, love, and a variety of spiritual ideals, I believe they all represent what my Higher Power wants me to have: God's will for me.

Today, prayers are my connection to the God *of my understanding.*

May you live as long as you wish
and love as long as you live.
—Robert A. Heinlein

I love how we come together and support each other's' recovery. I am so happy that recovery is possible, and that I don't have to do it alone. I love it that we can work together to help the still suffering nicotine addict. It's important to me that our meetings are a safe place to share from the heart, offering acceptance, support, and hope.

I love how I feel when I breathe in fresh air, and my lungs expand to let in the good oxygen I need. It feels so good to exert energy and then rest.

I love that I can feel the breeze sweep my cheeks with cold at the same time the sun blushes them with warmth. I get great joy from smelling a rose and tasting fresh food.

I love how I get the lessons I need at just the right time, to help me grow emotionally, mentally, spiritually. My Higher Power is there for me constantly, all I have to do is reach out.

Today, I find many ways to love life
and be present in this moment.

NOVEMBER 14

Let breath be my tether whenever there's stormy weather.
—Nicotine Anonymous Member

As a longtime member of another 12-Step fellowship, I began attending NicA meetings to get free of nicotine. However, each time I got closer to a quit date, my anxiety got harder to deal with and my resolve waned. Just the anticipation of letting go of nicotine left me feeling abandoned and disconnected. Clearly, I needed to be willing to do more if I was ever going to get free.

I began using the phone to connect with members, especially with another newcomer who also was struggling. Then, the two of us agreed to go to a retreat spa, and there we began our freedom from nicotine.

Despite the connections I was building in recovery, I still struggled with feeling untethered, because my constant companion was gone. So, I added other types of recovery meetings and activities to support my quit. I accepted I needed to be willing to go to any length.

I continued participating in this special kind of self-created retreat that provided simple sanity and healthy food. My connection with the breath grew ever more profound, as I found that breath is the connection with all living beings—the thread that links past, present, and future. As long as I make conscious contact with my breath, I am connected, I am tethered to life.

Today, I continue with my recovery process, one breath at a time.

Every problem is a character-building opportunity,
and the more difficult it is, the greater the potential
for building spiritual muscle and moral fiber.

—Rick Warren

As a child I was taught to believe in God, but then abandoned any notions of that kind of belief system. When I came into the program, I was spiritually bankrupt. But gradually, I became certain the only way to recover from this addiction was to let it go to some entity powerful enough to enable me to not take the addiction back no matter what—a Power greater than myself.

It was suggested I act as if I already had a Higher Power and to nurture this concept by committing to daily prayer. I read about others who had a strong spiritual practice, explored the creative beauty in nature, and served others in need.

Through discipline, time and attention, my own spirituality, and personal relationship with my Higher Power evolved. I learned if we treat ourselves and others with love and respect, spirituality grows.

The greatest gift from Nicotine Anonymous is my relationship with my Higher Power. There would be no recovery, no joy of living, no freedom from fear without it. Every day I thank God for being able to thank God.

Today, I will actively feed and exercise my spiritual muscles to keep them fit.

Don't seek for everything to happen as you wish it would,
but rather wish that everything happens as it actually will—
then your life will be serene.

—Epictetus

When I try to force my will on situations, I get frustrated because I cannot control others. Often when my expectations are not met, I feel uncomfortable, lose my serenity, and jeopardize my cherished freedom from nicotine.

When I pray for the guidance from my Higher Power, I surrender the things I cannot control. I cannot control other people or how others will respond. But I can control how I respond. I can take control of my own reactions to what is going on around me and to my own feelings. I can listen for knowledge of my Higher Power's will for me and ask for the power to carry that out.

It's like when I was quitting the use of nicotine. Instead of fighting cravings, I simply felt the craving, but I didn't act on it. I surrendered and focused on the prizes: my serenity and my freedom.

Today, I say the Serenity Prayer, breathe deeply, and let it go.

NOVEMBER 17

As this relationship with my Higher Power grows,
so am I, and my contentment, serenity,
and appreciation grows as well.
—Nicotine Anonymous Member

I like the idea of exercising my faith muscle. The God of my understanding and I have this growing relationship. We communicate with each other often, and my Higher Power shows up in ever-amazing ways in my life.

Sometimes I imagine wrapping my Higher Power's safe and loving arms around me and all is well. I surrender like I'm falling back into a warm, soft, cozy place. When I finally let go of control of what I cannot change, I holler for help, just as I would to a friend, "Hey, HP, I need your help!" When I'm really quiet and really listen, I sense what my Higher Power is saying. It's like a peaceful, inner knowing, a spaciousness in my heart, the small voice that's always there.

When I hear some kind of meaningful wisdom in a meeting, a synchronicity, or apparent goodness, happens out of nowhere, and I see that HP has communicated with me again. When I am thankful for all the abundance, I'm right there in the moment, breathing along with that Power greater than me, and finding more goodness keeps coming. My contentment grows, I am clean and serene.

Today, I am improving my conscious contact
with my Higher Power as I reach out to my Higher Power
and allow myself to be helped, nurtured, and loved.

NOVEMBER 18

"Sought through prayer and meditation
to improve our conscious contact with God..."
—Step Eleven

I pray: God, I ask for the serenity to live in harmony with my own essential nature. May Thy will be done, not mine. Guide and direct my thinking. Grant me willingness, courage, and strength through my actions, so that I may reflect your love and wisdom. Show me ways to serve my fellow members. Give me the willingness to let go of barriers and to fully live this life.

Inspire me with the splendor and majesty of the oceans, the rain, the sun, the stars, the mountains, the sky, the air, the flowers, and all the wonders you have created.

As I claim my freedom from the endless spiral of self-destruction, give me the wisdom to keep choosing the gift of my new life. Help me experience joy and happiness, today, here and now.

Today, I maintain and enjoy my recovery
through conversations with my Higher Power.

I hear medicine at meetings.
That's where I get my prescription filled.
—Nicotine Anonymous Member

My NicA meeting is my safe space, an oasis of support and sanity. Wealthy folks may have their expensive health spas, but I have my weekly NicA meeting for a buck or two donation. There, I get to pour out my experience, strength, and hope. Gratefully, I hear others' wisdom not yet found in my own head.

Meetings are where my heart is nourished and spirit is refreshed. My group practices the doctors' credo, "First, do no harm," by offering our mutual respect. Our format asks that members avoid crosstalk, which is how "we focus on ourselves and we do not interrupt, criticize, or offer unsolicited advice directly toward another member when they share."

I haven't always experienced this kind of safety outside of meetings. With this mutual respect, I'm not only more comfortable to speak my truth, but I also listen with a more open mind. Sometimes the best thing we do for one another is to do nothing but listen respectfully.

In so many ways, nicotine had me wandering in a desert of addiction. The Steps provide a pathway to recovery and a spiritual awakening. I spent years in my illness. I hope to spend my remaining years in my healing place.

Today, I keep my appointment with my Higher Doctor
in order to get my daily prescription filled.

When you come to the end of your rope, tie a knot and hang on.
— Franklin D. Roosevelt

I still have times when I feel overwhelmed by my life's daily events and momentarily think I have no alternative but to smoke a cigarette. So far, that thought is followed by, "But there is so much to lose."

Because of the NicA literature and my fellow members, I know more about the Tools and principles of recovery today, than when my brain was clouded with smoke. Now, I have many other alternatives to reach for, and a process I can trust.

I've been working our Steps using our *Nicotine Anonymous Step Study Workbook* with my sponsor. I've come to believe I can be restored to sanity. I have come to believe that all that nicotine I burned into my body was not my best friend.

I have come to believe that I am my own best friend. And now I have a group of better friends who I can hang on to when I feel overwhelmed, friends who help lift my spirits. Clearly, they are better than the pack of lies I once believed in.

I also realize I have alternatives as I come to my own understanding of a Power greater than myself. I'm committed to improving my conscious contact with this Power to keep my heart connected to my brain.

Today, as I enjoy another day of freedom from nicotine,
I am grateful for the Grace that restores me to sanity.

Tiny elements of matter operating collectively
become more than themselves,
to enable the cosmos to know itself.
—Neil DeGrasse Tyson

In his wisdom, Aristotle once wrote, "The whole is greater than the sum of its parts." Coaches use the T.E.A.M. acronym: Together, Everyone Achieves More. Nicotine Anonymous says it's a WE program. I believe our individual members also operate collectively and become more than themselves to enable the fellowship to know itself. Our primary purpose is in sync with this concept of synergy. That's a reason I came to believe NicA is a Power greater than myself.

Prior to joining our fellowship, I was not a club joiner. Clubs made individuals conform to their rules or shut out anyone not fitting some set standard. However, from the start in NicA I was told to take what I like and leave the rest, and that the Steps are suggestions. Tradition Two states, "Our leaders are but trusted servants; they do not govern." In "Our Policy of Openness" pamphlet it states, "...each member is free to come to their own understanding of a Power greater than themselves..."

My freedom from nicotine came when finally, I unconditionally surrendered. My way had been no way. Now, turning over my struggles to the collective power of our fellowship gives me the peace I seek. What relief!

Today, I meditate on improving
my conscious connection to the collective spirit.

NOVEMBER 22

With nicotine, it was my way or the highway, buddy!
—Nicotine Anonymous Member

Prior to joining NicA, my mantra was, "No one best get between me and my nicotine and don't bug me about it." Nicotine was my one drug of choice, and I didn't want to admit to myself or others my inner truth. I knew I was on the road to a painful disease. I just didn't know any alternatives until I found NicA.

Freedom started with admitting my secret desire to stop using nicotine. At meetings, I learned that instead of struggling, I could surrender and accept temporary discomforts. I had previously heard the adage, "This too shall pass." Now, I can apply that to cravings.

Rather than feeling doomed by this addiction, I make conscious contact with the care of a Power greater than myself. Instead of white knuckling to grasp willpower, I read in *Nicotine Anonymous: The Book* to seek the will of my Higher Power.

Instead of isolating in shame, I connect with members and a sponsor. Instead of being up to no good for myself, I do good for our fellowship. I have alternatives to nicotine that actually take care of what I truly need. I have a path that frees me of the bondage of self, and from nicotine.

Today, I will practice NicA principles
as a way to realize my freedom
and to carry the message of hope to others.

NOVEMBER 23

Still waters run deep.

—Latin proverb

My addiction thrived on chaos. When I had free time and did not know what to do, I would use nicotine. When I wanted to procrastinate, I would use some more. I would smoke when I woke up, went to sleep, needed to perk myself up, calm down, or suppress a feeling. I used nicotine before and after almost everything I did.

It wasn't until I put the nicotine down that I could see how much my addiction separated me from myself, my Higher Power, and from others. I came to realize there is no answer or strength in using nicotine in any form.

I find comfort and wisdom in those moments when I can slow down and just breathe. I stay quiet and still with my soul, God, and the universe. That is the time when the answers I need come to me. It is when I am quiet and still that I make a deep connection within myself and my Higher Power. It is when I focus, breathe, and listen that I hear the answers I seek. When I feel peaceful with a choice, I believe that choice is God's will for me. I live my life much more calmly and serenely now, which is what I wanted all along.

Today, I turn to God for the wisdom and serenity I seek.

NOVEMBER 24

Working the Steps of recovery is like a job with benefits.
—Nicotine Anonymous Member

I accept both the need and the value of working my program one day at a time. My life can be a lot to manage, so it has been helpful to only focus on a measured amount of time and activities. When I get overwhelmed, all I need to do is the next right thing. Also, I value sanity when I live in the present moment and avoid getting ahead of myself with a head full of anxiety.

Recovery is an ongoing responsibility. The efforts reward me with integrity, gratitude, confidence, and an inner oasis where I can find self-soothing serenity. There, I have no desire to use nicotine to escape, avoid, or numb myself. This responsibility improves my ability to respond to both the treasures and troubles of living with acceptance and courage. Daily conscious contact with my Higher Power offers experiences in recovery and develops inner wisdom. Attending NicA meetings regularly keeps me grounded and recharges my commitment to myself and my recovery.

Five days a week, I have a salaried avocation that pays my bills. Every day, I have my recovery vocation where I turn my will over to Good Orderly Direction.

Today, I gratefully receive the benefits gained from my recovery.

NOVEMBER 25

It is useful to remember that finding an understanding of a Higher Power is a process, not an event.

—Nicotine Anonymous: The Book

I was my own Higher Power. I didn't trust in God, but I was aware of a Power greater than me. While young, I thought of God as a punishing kind of god. As I grew older, I understood there are reasons for what happens in our lives, and that what happened to me was not about punishment at all.

Even as I understood this, I constantly tried being in the front seat, thinking I could control other people's feelings and control my own nicotine addiction. I didn't need anyone's help, and surely not God's to stop smoking. I told myself I could cut down or stop if I chose to.

I tried all the many ways to get a quit for years, thinking my use of nicotine was not an addiction. I just liked to use it. Yet the constant use of nicotine controlled my life, and my life was out of control.

Admitting I needed help was yet another hurdle for me to overcome. I felt it would be weak to accept help from someone else. Shouldn't I be helping others? Becoming humble took some time before I accepted help and understood it was okay to allow others to help me.

Now in recovery, I reach out to my Higher Power, my sponsor and others when I need help. I learned that asking for help is a humbling experience.

Today, God steers and I enjoy the ride
from the passenger's seat.

NOVEMBER 26

Illness begins with I; Wellness begins with We.
—Swami Satchidananda

Before finding Nicotine Anonymous, I thought of myself as one person alone with my problem, my nicotine use. I'd heard of nicotine cessation groups that lasted a few weeks with tricks like snapping a rubber band on the wrist each time the urge to use nicotine came up. I knew I would just have one heck of a sore wrist as I used up my stash. I couldn't conceive of how other people could help me stop using, short of locking me in a padded cell.

Tradition One states, "Our common welfare should come first; personal recovery depends upon Nicotine Anonymous unity." Alone, I was stuck in my disease and my personal shortcomings. Through my connection to members, working the Steps, and using our Tools of recovery, I have found the medicines that have eased my disease and inspired me to be the person I want to be.

Nicotine Anonymous: The Book says, "Individually, we are one for all, as a group we are all for one." I found a safe place where I could receive healing, as well as give to others the gifts I have been so freely given.

Today, I will practice mutual support and keep growing through the process of recovery.

NOVEMBER 27

Cigarettes, like wolves, travel in packs.
—Nicotine Anonymous Member

At first, cigarettes followed me everywhere like a pet dog, a constant companion. I was mostly in denial about the damage each cigarette caused me physically, emotionally, and spiritually. Any gaps in denial were filled with excuses.

Inevitably, my dog began to bark and nip at me until the dog became a howling and biting wolf. Then, packs of cigarettes became a pack of wolves. I had chest pains, shortness of breath, and smoking-related illnesses. On my own, I continually felt like prey being hunted down by nicotine predators.

Joining a Nicotine Anonymous meeting, I found a pack of members to rely on for support. Then I learned I had a pack of changes to begin making in my behavior and attitudes. That was scary, and at first, I resisted working some of the Twelve Steps.

However, NicA is a gentle program. My fellow members created a safe and inspiring place to make the changes I needed to gain the benefits of living without nicotine. Now, I'm no longer prey. Instead, I pray.

Today, my pack of NicA Tools helps me maintain vigilance against the wolf pack's return.

NOVEMBER 28

Faith is the complete reliance
on the power and goodness of Spirit
and the firm belief that you are always connected
to this goodness. Always affirm your faith and not your doubt.
—Wayne Dwyer

When I'm anxious, I'm in fear. For me, most fear originates from self- doubt and a terror of being alone, abandoned and forsaken. I've had to climb out of that dark hole of fear and realize I am not alone, and that no matter what, there are those around me who love and support me.

Fear can feed the cycle of stinking thinking and using nicotine, which feeds the power my addiction has over me. I have admitted that I am unable to stop the cycle on my own.

Faith is believing in the goodness of the God of my understanding, and that I am no longer alone. A power much greater than myself is always there for me unconditionally. When I have an open mind, I'm available to my relationship with my Higher Power. I am able to trust this Great Spirit, to trust myself, and to be present with myself, with others, and with this Power greater than me.

I make progress, not perfection. But because **Smoking is Not an Option**, I get to focus on what really matters to me, what I really want to spend my energy on. I make choices to be happy and feel good.

Today, I am shown the way of honesty, openness, and willingness;
I believe I am loved and supported.

NOVEMBER 29

Recovery is an "inside job."
—Nicotine Anonymous Member

As a nicotine addict, I was fixated on using something that was outside me to make something happen inside me. I used nicotine to filter the outside world so I might feel better. I realize now that was a plan doomed to eventual frustration and failure for myself, and that it also hurt others.

I read the pamphlet, "How Nicotine Anonymous Works" to understand how healing can come from the inside with honesty, open mindedness, and willingness. I'm changing my life experience by focusing on changing myself, not other people, places, and things. My life is better, and that works out better for others.

I cannot rearrange life so that it is without problems, frustrations, or pain. However, by changing HOW I respond to life, I can directly affect my experience. I have the Serenity Prayer. I cannot change the power of nicotine, but I can change how I behave. I cannot hold the wind, but I can learn to breathe and have peace of mind.

Today, I focus on my inner self and this program's principles, because that's HOW it works.

NOVEMBER 30

What I needed was a connection to life
that was real and lasting.
—Claire Danes

Initially, I used nicotine to feel pleasure and appear cool. For a time, it seemed successful. Eventually it became clear that using nicotine was mainly to avoid feeling uncomfortable, and there was nothing cool about it. Using it just relieved the awful withdrawal symptoms.

With the support and recovery resources from my Nicotine Anonymous group, I finally became willing to go through the challenge of withdrawal to gain my freedom. For a while, I would have cravings for nicotine along with feeling a sense of loss that something was missing. I accepted those feelings, not as cravings, but as memories of how I reacted in the past to various triggers. It was clear I was having moments, not of a chemical crave, but of an actual human need for a connection to life.

Sometimes, the feeling of need came at an awkward lull between ordinary, or even pleasurable, activities. Momentarily, I was at a loss to know what to do with myself. My sponsor suggested those could be moments to take a deep breath, be grateful, or make conscious contact with my Higher Power. They could be spiritual opportunities to pause and connect, or just smile at the mystery of the moment.

Today, I seek spiritual fulfillment through opportunities to connect with what is real and lasting.

DECEMBER 1

Having had a spiritual awakening as the result of these Steps,
We tried to carry this message to nicotine users,
and practice these principles in all our affairs.
—Step Twelve

Hearing about a Nicotine Anonymous meeting, I felt pulled toward it. If someone had pushed me, I would have resisted. I wasn't ready then to stop using nicotine. I appreciated how Tradition Three meant that it wasn't a requirement to have quit, and that helped me to feel welcome. I only needed my one truth, a desire to gain my independence from nicotine. I wanted my inalienable rights to life, liberty, and the pursuit of happiness.

The maturity I gained in recovery made it clear that such rights come with responsibilities. The Twelve Steps and Twelve Traditions are my list of responsibilities in order to gain the right to live free and happy. As I continue to take care of my responsibilities and practice these principles in all my affairs, I continue to enjoy these rights.

I am grateful for our Twelve Steps' guidance that has brought me to a spiritual awakening. Step Twelve encourages me to carry the message of recovery to others still suffering from this insidious addiction. In doing so, shame is lifted from when I spewed toxins at others. And Tradition Eleven adds its guidance. When carrying the message, my actions ought to be based on attraction rather than promotion, because it's my actions that speak louder than what I say.

Today, I offer my service as my response for being liberated.

DECEMBER 2

Anonymity is the spiritual foundation of all our Traditions,
ever reminding us to place principles before personalities.
—Tradition Twelve

My first home group, in a small town, contained a wide variety of personalities. Over the years, I've attended other groups, intergroup retreats, and numerous World Services Conferences. I've been a board member and served as a coordinator. Oh, the personalities! Keeping program principles in place is our saving grace, even when not always handled gracefully. It's often joked, "Everyone has an opinion."

Traditions One, Three, and Five are anchors, especially for service work. These words of wisdom guide my actions and attitudes: "our common welfare," "the only requirement," and "one primary purpose."

I find the Traditions are helpful outside the meeting rooms. My home and professional life improve when I'm mindful of what is in the best interest for our common welfare. My only requirement is a desire to be relieved of the bondage of self and to do good in this world and show kindness. Step Twelve guides me to practice these principles in all my affairs. With Grace's mercy, I'm guided to humbly seek progress not perfection.

Today, for our common welfare, I pray for all,
and ask that they be granted the same peace that I seek.

DECEMBER 3

Nothing ever goes away until it teaches us
what we need to know.
—Pema Chodron

My mind is where my disease resides. I have a thinking disease. I need to remember this so when those pesky addictive thoughts come in, I can use the Tools and Twelve Steps available to me in my spiritual toolkit.

I start with the first three Steps, a foundation that needs to be strong or the rest will collapse. "I can't, He can, so I'll let Him." I say that simple prayer to myself every morning to remind me that I am not in charge.

The Fourth through the Ninth Steps are action Steps to help me clean house and straighten up the destruction of the past. Steps Ten through Twelve are my growing Steps, which teach me that my purpose is to serve others. They are the roof on the Twelve Step structure that will help me stay safe and warm as long as I keep it in good repair.

Along this spiritual path, as I am learning to live life on life's terms, I notice pesky thoughts before acting on them, and move on to better feelings and thoughts. I get the lessons I need exactly when I need them, and use my spiritual toolkit to guide my actions.

Today, I am deeply grateful for all that has been given to me,
all that has fallen away,
and the abundance of goodness that remains.

DECEMBER 4

What is more mortifying than to feel
that you have missed the plum
for want of courage to shake the tree?
—Logan Pearsall Smith

For the last fifteen years of my smoking, I dreaded the reality that someday my family would have to watch me die due to my addiction. I couldn't blame it on ignorance. I didn't argue with science. Reality was slapping me in the face with nearly every cigarette I stuck in my mouth. This took a toll on my self-esteem and on my ability to feel empowered to move forward in my life. On my own, I could not find the courage to deal with the cravings.

Now, I am staying clean from nicotine one day at a time. I am deeply grateful to our fellowship for my freedom. This gratitude gives me courage to offer service. As I practice the Twelfth Step, whether by doing service or carrying the message to nicotine users, I am given an opportunity to recover my self-esteem. Now, I feel that I truly have something of value to offer others who desire to live nicotine free.

While I carry the message and do service, it feels like I am sowing seeds. As my efforts bear fruit, I reap the reward of feeling more courage to continue expanding the ways I can serve. In order to keep my freedom, I must practice the principles on a daily basis. I've come to believe that this program works if I work it.

Today, I receive the grace of courage
to shake off my fear of inadequacy
and harvest the fruits of my recovery.

DECEMBER 5

When the fear of remaining the same
overcomes the fear of change, recovery is possible.
Everything will fail until I am prepared
to do all that is necessary to succeed.
—Nicotine Anonymous Member

An amazing sense of calm during a crisis is one of the greatest gifts of recovery that freedom from nicotine has given to me. I am no longer adding nicotine withdrawal on top of every stressful event. I've been awarded inner peace and happiness, which are all I've ever really wanted.

I was one of those people who sleep-walked through life. I didn't think about who I was or what I wanted to be. Then one day, I woke up and wondered why I was unhappy. I saw this as an opportunity for change.

My addiction is one of the best things that ever happened to me. My addiction moved me to change and find an inner peace and tranquility. I find recovery rewarding because I get the chance to change my life, come to know my Higher Power, and help others.

People in recovery often describe themselves as grateful addicts. There are few places in the world where I find more honesty, courage, and support than in a Twelve Step meeting. Gratefully, ours is a spiritual approach to a spiritual problem arising from addiction.

My freedom from nicotine is the single most important thing in my life. If anything jeopardizes that, it's eliminated. Recovery and the Twelve Steps have changed my life. I will never take this freedom for granted.

Today, my spiritual awakening has me believe in miracles,
because I am one.

DECEMBER 6

Wellness means I am okay.
Spirituality leads to We are okay.
—Sarah Bowen

Addiction made me self-centered each time I used nicotine. It was an isolated state walled off from reality and separated from others. Fears and feelings of inadequacy that began in my youth had remained an undercurrent in my adult life.

For me to be *okay* and have wellness, I needed to become honest, open, and willing. That's how Nicotine Anonymous works. I used the five Tools and answered the questions in the *Step Study Workbook*. I recited the Serenity Prayer often to ask for acceptance, courage, and wisdom. These resources were the medicine that got me well, living free of nicotine, and restoring me to sanity.

I developed trustworthy connections with my Higher Power and my fellow members, and offered acts of service in various ways to the fellowship. These actions led me to a spiritual awakening that was a healing transformation.

Spirituality, in my understanding, is about connecting to life in all its forms and offering acts of kindness and care.

Today, as I continue to heal, I connect to the spiritual We, and practice the principles that have freed me.

DECEMBER 7

Get present with where you are and what is happening
in order to get where you want to be.
—Anonymous

I started attending meetings and was willing to hear what other members had to say. I found I was like many others who had tried everything to quit but nothing had worked. I was desperate to quit, but I didn't believe that my miracle was waiting for me.

I kept showing up at meetings, found a sponsor, shared honestly where I was in my recovery, worked the Steps and Traditions, allowed others to help, and used the Tools of the program. The first three Steps were vitally important in my recovery. They showed me I am truly powerless over nicotine, that my life had become unmanageable and that I needed a Power greater than myself to restore me to sanity.

I am incredibly grateful for the powerful principles of this program and for all those who walked before me and beside me. This has helped me overcome my addiction to nicotine. As a result, I have many years of freedom from nicotine, practicing the principles in all my affairs one day at a time.

Today, from this present moment forward,
I thank my Higher Power for showing me
how to live in the process of recovery.

DECEMBER 8

I started getting my quit
when I started giving to others.
—Nicotine Anonymous Member

When I entered my first NicA meeting I was looking to get something that would make me stop using nicotine. Meeting after meeting, I kept wondering when I would get it.

A founding member of the group asked me if I would consider the service of opening the door each week. I paused while thinking, "Hey, I'm here to get something from the group, not do something for them." But that felt like a rude attitude, so I said that I would. Although I was still using nicotine, I now felt I had some value. Eventually, I realized how that request opened the door to my recovery.

For many years I have offered service in various ways, including sponsoring members who came through that meeting door. I remain mindful that being open to serve is how I've gotten so much more than I had originally sought. I could not get until I gave.

Getting and giving happens by keeping my own door open. It's how we humans breathe and learn. Getting and giving is an indivisible relationship. Just as my exhale and inhale are necessary for either to be effective, I can't have one without the other.

Today, I will keep my door open
to give and get what I need.

DECEMBER 9

Time is going to pass anyway, so, I'd rather
be where I want to be, than where I could've been.
—Carl Alamby

Carl's story was a televised segment about fortitude. He grew up in an impoverished neighborhood. He had dreams of being a doctor, but that didn't seem realistic. So, he got practical and settled for being an excellent mechanic. Carl worked hard on cars in a parking lot. He saved up, got his own shop, and became a respected master mechanic. Nearly 40, Carl enrolled in college to get a business degree, but one biology class was required.

Instantly, he was inspired to pursue his dream. He set a course for the next nine years to become a doctor. His friends questioned why he would now give up the next nine years of his life. His answer was the quote above. He has become a well-respected emergency room doctor.

For 20 years, I dreamed of quitting smoking. When I joined Nicotine Anonymous, I didn't know what to expect. Soon, I unexpectedly became willing to be a trusted servant. Over many years, I've served in various positions. Friends also wondered how many years I would keep focusing on Nicotine Anonymous rather than nicotine. I didn't have a plan quite like Carl, but with the fortitude and commitment I gained, I have accomplishments beyond my wildest dreams.

---

*Today, I'm grateful I invested the time to recover and
to be where I want to be, rather than where I could've been.*

DECEMBER 10

I can't get no satisfaction.
'Cause I try and I try and I try and I try.
—Keith Richards, Mick Jagger

College was the beginning of my many unsuccessful attempts to stop smoking. Out of money and mind, I dropped out in my third year. Life went on with its cycles of ups and lasting downs for 20 more years. Days would often end feeling I hadn't done enough. I just couldn't access a full deep sense of satisfaction. It was the same with nicotine. No matter how many hits, it seemed never enough. There was no lasting satisfaction, just a temporary drug-induced stupor.

The Steps and meetings have given me many insights. I've realized I used nicotine to numb the enduring dissatisfactions I felt. I had lived with a general sense of something missing or not enough. Ongoing meetings gave me time, a safe place, and a program of hope until I let go and got free.

Filling the emptiness with service in NicA gives me purpose and satisfaction. My deepening gratitude connects me to those I care about and to all I have gained. Recovery restored me with a new confidence to return to college and get a master's degree. My willingness to work on my own program of recovery has resulted in a spiritual awakening, the essential part of what was missing in my life.

Today, I access my desire for satisfaction by practicing the principles of the program in all my affairs.

DECEMBER 11

Each group should be autonomous
except in matters affecting other groups
or Nicotine Anonymous as a whole.
—Tradition Four

Among the sources of stress that I used to rationalize my need for nicotine, were my spouse, my children, and people at my job. There were issues of control and change that caused tension among us. At times, there was an attitude of my way or the highway. Discussions became arguments, as if we were lawyers out to win our case. Without resolution, my spouse and I would ask for a continuance, and separate to use nicotine. My children watched us use nicotine and learned to act like lawyers themselves.

The Steps guided my spouse and me to gain freedom from nicotine. The Traditions guided us on how to better interact with others. We created a safe atmosphere to listen respectfully, accept differences, consider new ideas, seek solutions rather than victories. We remained mindful of how any decisions impacted our family as a whole. I also improved how I interacted with my work mates.

If we are both to remain happy, joyous, and free, we've decided to use the Steps and Traditions and practice these principles in all our affairs. The positive effect this has on our children shows us that it works if we all work it.

*Today, I pray that my family be granted
the same peace that I seek.*

I celebrate a month nicotine free,
but at times I'm free falling, hoping for a parachute.
—Nicotine Anonymous Member

Hearing a member share this brought me back to my first nicotine-free month, when I was both excited and still rather disoriented. It had taken many months of attending my NicA meeting before I finally ventured into my first hours of freedom from nicotine. I had felt embarrassed to show up because I was still using nicotine. However, my group members always put me at ease with their support and acceptance.

Hindsight often provides a clearer understanding of experiences; if lessons are sought, they are often highly revealing. Once I began to be restored to sanity, I realized the benefit of those many months of attending meetings while I was still using nicotine. I had time to develop connections with other members, to develop trust, and to feel safe among peers. I had time for them to become my parachute whenever I felt I was free falling.

I'm aware that parachutes must be packed by a person who is certified and follows specific steps. NicA has specific Steps and Traditions based on spiritual and moral principles that guide each member. We have the protection of anonymity and confidentiality regarding who and what is shared and heard. NicA continues to safely land me on my feet, one day at a time.

Today, I venture forth with confidence,
knowing I always have a parachute.

DECEMBER 13

No matter what it is, it's never enough.
—Nicotine Anonymous Member

Only sleep could end my daily doses of nicotine. I always cleaned my plate and sought seconds. My curiosity had endless questions. When it came to ingesting things, craving more was a state of mind. I wanted more, often until it hurt. Even at my job, I worked at tasks until I was exhausted. I couldn't recognize or accept when I had done enough, much less that I was enough.

At NicA meetings I heard others who had similar behaviors in addition to our nicotine-driven behavior. Was I an insatiable abyss like a black hole, or was I missing what could actually satisfy me? Nicotine addiction brought me into the program, but recovering into a new serene and satisfying life would require my full use of the Steps and Tools. I needed to be willing to go to any length. I was used to going to limitless lengths for nicotine, but now in the program, I had Good Orderly Direction.

In NicA I am receiving caring support, and I am giving of myself in service. My weekly meetings are fulfilling. I am a work in progress and my tomorrows have more for me to do. Yet for today, I am enough.

Today, I continue my journey in recovery
with serenity and satisfaction.

DECEMBER 14

Our spiritual life is not a theory, we have to live it.
—"Our Promises"

What does it mean to live a spiritual life? How can a hard-core nicotine addict turn things around and live life on a spiritual basis?

For me, it has been a gradual process. As the smokescreen cleared around me and inside me, I began to notice little things, obvious things that before quitting, I wasn't present enough to notice. It was like awakening from a long sleep to find new sounds, smells, and sights everywhere.

Working the Steps added still more dimension and the awareness that I don't live in isolation, that everything I do and say affects others. Even what I think has an effect. I realized my Higher Power was showing me the connectedness of all things, and that although I am but one, I must strive to be the best one I can be.

That's how I came to see how much I need this program. Left to my own devices, such an enterprise would falter and fail. But because of the meetings, the literature, and the Steps, I am continuously made aware of the principles I must live by. Thanks to my Higher Power, a life of smoking and shutting others out has been replaced by a willingness to engage, to be a part of, and to come from a spiritual place to the best of my ability.

Today, to stay free, I live a spiritual life in the Nicotine Anonymous program.

DECEMBER 15

Burdens are sometimes blessings in disguise.
—Steve Hartman

My first reaction to doing acts of service was that it would be a burden, a responsibility. I equated freedom to being able to avoid any unnecessary responsibilities. I didn't want to burden my precious time or fragile emotions with distractions that kept me from my preferred pleasure-seeking activities.

However, as my gratitude grew for the support of my group's members, I came to believe that service was my gratitude in action. There was a sanity to service in how it became a balancing of goodness between what I gained and what I could give, a healing for what had hurt.

I accepted and initiated ways to serve my group, and then World Services. The projects and personalities involved have surely been a challenge. I placed principles over personalities so I could improve my patience and persistence. I am willing to have my lack of a skill exposed, be humble and yet assertive, and mostly not have everything my way. I learned to manage my life, to mature emotionally, to address challenges, and to be relieved of the bondage of self. Now my service is to help those who are suffering. Service is a blessing, which starts by focusing on Nicotine Anonymous rather than nicotine.

Today, I ask that any sense of burden be lifted
by focusing on all I've gained through service.

DECEMBER 16

When I started smoking as a kid, I was trying to be a big show off.
But my recovery has been about being a big show up.
—Nicotine Anonymous Member

A group member recently said to me, "You're a big show up," acknowledging how I **Keep Showing Up** at one, two, or three meetings a week, and have for more than 30 years.

I practice our slogan, **First Aid First**. I go to meetings because "Our Promises" remind me that, "We begin to forget we had been nicotine users, except at meetings." Living nicotine free for so many years is the result of showing up at meetings. I don't ever want to think that nicotine is the solution. Clearly, my addictive thinking is the problem.

At my very first NicA meeting there were members who had gotten free. Their showing up showed me it was possible and gave me hope. I **Keep Showing Up** to give back what I have been given: support and wisdom gained from all members, past and present. Even more than just coming back, it's important to *show up* and show that *it works if you work it.*

Today, I remain committed to carry the message
and show the gift of recovery to others.

DECEMBER 17

Our victory over our own difficulties encouraged us to continue, and we became an example for others as well.

—*Nicotine Anonymous: The Book*

As a newcomer, I thought I had nothing to give toward service. Then after hearing some people in the meeting explain that service could be just showing up to a meeting, I felt relieved. I saw recovery in action as I watched other members help out during meetings, reach out to newcomers, or step up for a service position.

By my second month clean from nicotine, I read the Steps or Traditions in meetings. I shared my experience, strength and hope, and did whatever I could to participate. By my ninth month, I co-chaired a meeting and felt great joy in my heart as members showed their appreciation.

Finally, I felt like I belonged to this group of people who knew what I was going through. I was accepted and supported, and wanted to contribute as best as I could in my own time. The more I immersed myself in my own recovery, the more my quit was supported. By stepping up for service, I show that I am blessed with a new freedom and a new happiness, and that "Our Promises" are coming true.

Today, I practice NicA principles with those in my life as well as in the fellowship.

DECEMBER 18

Abundance flows freely through me.

—Louise Hay

I spent years addicted to nicotine and living with negative thoughts about myself and my life. To improve my self-esteem, I affirm the positive in me and my life. Affirmations are healing messages that I send myself each day. I use affirmations to pump joy into my heart through these healing messages.

When I choose to affirm the good in myself and life, I break the chains of stinking thinking: the resentments, fears, and reactivity. Over time, using affirmations brings serenity and peace of mind.

Affirmations bring out the best of my real self and strengthen my spirit. The positive messages empower me to change my thinking. Although I am still powerless over nicotine, my spirituality grows through these affirming words.

For example, I affirm character assets such as I am filled with faith, I am loving and kind, I am trustworthy and trust myself, and I am a talented, beautiful person. Even during tough times, I detach from reacting to life's worries, and I am proactive about taking good care of myself.

My sponsor applauds when I am proactive instead of waiting until the middle of a disaster to take action. I can affirm myself into freedom from fear by saying that all is well, I am safe. I have become more self-confident and experience a real inner joy in my heart.

Today, I am enough, and I am worth it!

Meeting makers make it.
—Nicotine Anonymous Member

When I first showed up to witness recovery, I heard that truth. Some thought they could find an easier way. Others hung in there until they experienced a miracle in their life. They were living free from nicotine, and they hadn't gone completely crazy.

Surely, they had to get through some fog and confusion, yet these addicts in recovery kept showing up. Sometimes they got cranky, and still kept showing up. As difficult as it was for some, no one I knew died from quitting. We were reborn into a life free from nicotine's prison. It has been a beautiful thing to see again and again.

I've always been grateful to those who slipped but then returned to try again. There have been many who didn't return. When I see others smoking, I'm amazed that through my Higher Power's grace and my willingness, I haven't put a cigarette in my hand since I stopped. I recognize nicotine's power over me.

At meetings I experience the solution. The miracle of my recovery is a result of support from the fellowship, sanity from the Steps, and serenity from my Higher Power.

Today, a meeting is a time for me to be grateful that I have a place to celebrate my miracle.

DECEMBER 20

The best and most beautiful things in the world
cannot be seen or even touched—
they must be felt with the heart.
—Helen Keller

Because of my Higher Power, I have new joys I never have known or felt before. This program has brought me new hope. I can have or do anything in the whole Universe, except for nicotine. What infinite options I have to choose from!

For now, the best use of my time is to go to any length to keep from lighting up until I no longer think about using nicotine. I work the Steps. I also use the Tools by going to meetings, reading the literature, doing service, and connecting with my sponsor and members between meetings. I practice NicA principles, reach out to others and take good care of myself.

Thank you to those who have walked this path and carried the message before I arrived. Thanks for showing us newbies the way. Now it's my time to serve, my time to give back, to help the still suffering addicts so they can feel as incredibly good as I do today.

Today, I have new faith and hope as I feel joy in my recovery, one day at a time.

DECEMBER 21

To be a trusted servant,
it's helpful to read the Third Step Prayer which begins with,
"Relieve me of the bondage of self."
—Nicotine Anonymous Member

When I began offering to be of service, I soon realized the value and challenge of a WE program. My efforts had purpose, both for me and others. I could offer the skills I had, while others contributed the skills I lacked. Collaboration with others requires mutual agreement; it is a challenging practice to pray, "Relieve me of the bondage of self."

In our pamphlet, "How Nicotine Anonymous Works," I learn that being honest with oneself and others sometimes raises difficult feelings. While in service to others, I practice more humbly accepting any suggestions and perspectives offered when I remember how much I am learning from my fellow members.

Because personal recovery depends upon Nicotine Anonymous unity, I am grateful that we are a gentle program. At meetings, we practice mutual respect as we each share and listen. At business meetings, we practice faith in our group conscience as a Power greater than ourselves. These are among the ways we practice these principles in all our affairs.

I have faith in my group and in the care offered by a Power greater than myself. Surrendering to this caring trust keeps me focused on a higher purpose of service.

Today, I am guided by the Third Step Prayer
to inspire and direct my thinking.

DECEMBER 22

We come to believe in a Power greater than ourselves,
and then to serve a purpose greater than ourselves.
—Nicotine Anonymous Member

I had to come to NicA meetings before I could come to believe in a Power greater than me, a Power that could change me. I first arrived immersed in doubts that I could ever stop using nicotine. Years of failure had proven that. Yet with all my baggage, I was welcomed, accepted, supported, and given a home away from home.

My home group became a Power greater than my doubts and fears. My fellow members had succeeded in quitting and kept the meeting open for years so other nicotine addicts would find a home.

I was soon asked to set up the literature display. Fear wanted to say no, but gratitude said yes. That service got me to read all the literature. The literature became a powerful Tool I carried with me. Those words helped me stop vaping nicotine.

Accepting service has been a growth opportunity. It asks me to focus on our primary purpose rather than myself. Service continues to help raise my self-esteem, provide a means to make amends, and be an expression of my spiritual awakening.

Today, service carries our message and gives me a purpose greater than myself, giving back what I was given.

DECEMBER 23

My mission in life is not merely to survive, but to thrive;
and to do so with some passion, some compassion,
some humor, and some style.
—Maya Angelou

I have been given a life to live on this planet. And today, I celebrate being given back my life with freedom from nicotine. All I have is today to make it full of love, life, and laughter. It takes a new found attitude to come alive with grace and gusto rather than just getting by.

Take my creative work: because I feel stagnant and unfulfilled when I am not creating, I try to spend more time using my talents and skills to create things. I make this a priority. I prefer to thrive, loving what I do and doing what I love. I want to live my life to the fullest, creating amazing works, laughing, and having fun.

I avoid taking myself too seriously and often find humor in life's silliness and awe in life's wonder. I only need to remember to not pick up a cigarette no matter what. As a member of the No Matter What Club, now there is nothing holding me back.

Today, I live life to the fullest with a spirit
that continues to awaken and thrive.

DECEMBER 24

I sense a connection between the hole and the holy.
—Nicotine Anonymous Member

Joining Nicotine Anonymous, I heard members talk about the hole or, the hole in our soul. That described the bottomless pit and the emptiness that no amount of nicotine could truly satisfy, relieve distress, or bring comfort from relentless concerns. It's true that one is too many and a thousand are never enough.

After fearfully resisting for months, I finally let go of nicotine and more heartily held on to my group. Within weeks, I was beginning to feel relief from that gnaw in my craw. Although I felt better, the hole in my soul was not fully healed. I observed more seasoned members, and I wanted more of what they had. My sponsor encouraged me to keep working my program if I wanted the most out of my recovery. We started using our *Step Study Workbook*. My answers revealed more insights into my past, my present, and the path I wanted to take into a better life.

I still have work to do, especially on my resistance to let go, if I am to respect the gift of my recovery as something sacred and holy. To truly heal the hole in my soul and to have the peace I seek, my work is to seek a spiritual awakening through my relationship with a god of my own understanding.

Today, with each step forward in our program,
I am filled with more peace.

We must be willing to let go of the life we have planned,
so as to have the life that is waiting for us.
—E. M. Forster

I stopped smoking by working the Nicotine Anonymous program. My quit day was not a special day in particular, though it has certainly turned out to be. Each milestone has been a celebration of life. The gift is following the NicA spiritual path, which keeps me happily smober and able to meet life on life's terms. I didn't anticipate how wonderful my life in recovery would turn out to be, all because of my special quit day.

It takes such a leap of faith for us addicts to trust that our Higher Power will be there when we put down nicotine, will help us through it, and will bring us to the other side into freedom. Many aren't able to make that leap, and suffer greatly from the effects of this lethal addiction. I am thankful that something in me said, "Go for it. See what happens." It has meant the difference between a life of bondage and ill health, and one of freedom, growth, and grace.

I still go to weekly meetings, sponsor, and do other acts of service. This is how I express gratitude for what the God of my understanding has done, and continues to do for me. I give back to a program that showed me a better way and ultimately saved my life. I get the continual reminder that nicotine will kill me, that smoking doesn't really make anything better, and that HP has a better plan.

Today, I celebrate the new life I have chosen on this spiritual path with my friends in the program.

DECEMBER 26

When we are in our gratitude, we do not use nicotine.
—Newcomer's Booklet

Although gaining freedom from nicotine has been an essential part of my recovery, Nicotine Anonymous has given me so much more than a life free from nicotine. I have found, as the *Newcomer's Booklet* describes, that I "live more joyously with the clarity, humility, and gratitude the Step process provides." I am continually humbled with gratitude for how my life has transformed.

More than the toxic fog of this addiction has been lifted. The arrogant self-centeredness of the disease is replaced by humbly offering support and service. The daily unmanageability is exchanged for a spiritual awakening.

Living with gratitude is a gift in itself. Recovery has led to a deeper gratitude than I had ever known. Gratitude is more than an attitude. Gratitude is my peaceful refuge that restores my sanity during my daily endeavors. Gratitude becomes a spiritual state of being with which I want to continually improve my conscious contact. As I do, I experience how I am emotionally nourished and inspired to do good in this world.

Today, gratitude grants me the peace that I seek
and awakens my spirit each day.

Trust that they're making their lives work
in the way that they're making their lives work.
And just teach through the power of your example.
—Abraham Hicks

Sponsorship is a Tool of recovery. I learned that to keep the gift, we need to give it away, so I pay the gift forward to another member. Serving as a sponsor is one way to express my gratitude for the support and wisdom I received when I was welcomed at my first home group.

My efforts as a sponsor improve with both experience and the literature resources from World Services. I use the Questionnaire and the sections on the Twelve Steps in *Nicotine Anonymous: The Book*. The pamphlet, "How Nicotine Anonymous Works: Honesty, Openness, and Willingness," helps me keep mindful of those principles. The *Nicotine Anonymous Step Study Workbook* provides a hands-on method to work the Steps. We have a lot of resources to draw upon to enhance sponsorship relationships.

I use the guidance of the Third Step Prayer, "Show me the way of patience, tolerance, kindliness, and love" I create trust by honoring confidentiality. I consider NicA to be a gentle program, so avoid judgmental statements or criticisms. I listen rather than lecture. I want to stay attentive, so I share my experience, strength, and hope with the caveat, "Take what you like and leave the rest."

Today, I serve and use our many NicA resources
to practice the principles in all my affairs.

We now realize we have been participating in a grand hoax.
We haven't given up anything at all.
—"Our Promises"

The words I heard in my culture to describe the transformation of ending one's use of nicotine were typically stopping, quitting, and giving up. Those words only reinforced my anxiety about losing something if I no longer used nicotine. The very idea of having less for someone who couldn't get enough to fill whatever was missing felt like a no-win situation.

However, with the increasing nicotine-related health consequences, my list of excuses and rationalizations no longer worked. When I heard about a Nicotine Anonymous meeting, I decided to at least check it out, but made no promises. The meeting format included reading "Our Promises" aloud. I was struck by the words about the grand hoax. I was handed a Newcomer's Packet of literature that included the pamphlet, "Tips For Gaining Freedom From Nicotine." The next week the chairperson asked if anyone had a topic. I asked if it could be about what members gain by getting free from nicotine.

Using nicotine since I was a child, I didn't know what I was missing until I gained freedom from nicotine in NicA. I've found words can inspire a change of attitude and behavior. It's true, I promise!

Today, I read the words in our literature
for the truth and principles that inspire me.

DECEMBER 29

Man never has what he wants,
because what he wants is everything.
—C.-F. Ramuz

I am a creature of passions, which are sometimes tempered by reason. To successfully sail the adventurous seas of my desires requires learning healthy living skills and developing positive attitudes.

No matter at what stage I was, whether a child, an adolescent, or an adult, I wanted something. Coming to terms with my expectations about whether or not I got those things was an ongoing challenge.

I started using nicotine to get something I wanted. I wanted to appear to have the power of an adult and to be more accepted by my peers. And since I couldn't get everything I wanted, nicotine's numbing ability soothed my sense of deprivation. However, I became addicted, and the cravings kept me continually wanting more. I was in a perpetual cycle, obsessed, and out of control.

Now, as I work the Steps, I am having a spiritual awakening. I am becoming more fully awake and have come to believe that what I want is deeper and more profound than using nicotine.

Today, my spiritual journey fulfills me with a deep peace that nicotine could never provide.

DECEMBER 30

Nicotine Anonymous takes our lemons
and makes a lemonade stand.
—Nicotine Anonymous Member

I started with, "Why can't I quit when everyone else can?" Joining NicA, I came to believe I could gain and maintain freedom from nicotine because I was with others who desired the same. I believe Nicotine Anonymous takes in our experiences, develops them into strengths, and generates hope.

Our Nicotine Anonymous "Slogans" pamphlet says, "Your impossible becomes our possible as we each realize that together, we change." First, Nicotine Anonymous showed me how to change my lemons into lemonade. Then, our Tool of service showed me how I can volunteer to turn my lemonade into a lemonade stand. Service enables me to give back what I've been given. In a variety of ways, I am able to offer my experience, strength, and hope to other members. In the process, I grow as a person, make living amends, and explore new challenges I had been too afraid to attempt in the past.

NicA restores my life with worth and dignity. I'm happy I decided to serve my lemonade at our lemonade stand. I continue to be grateful for the opportunities that service gives me to discover my increasing potential as I recover my spiritual self.

Today, I find ways to serve as part of my daily spiritual nourishment.

DECEMBER 31

Don't Look to Graduate
—Nicotine Anonymous Slogan

When I first joined NicA in my hometown, I doubted it could somehow help me stop smoking. After all, I hadn't been able to do so on my own for many years. After several months of attending meetings and still smoking, I wondered, "How long am I going to have to attend meetings to get what others got?" Gratefully, I kept showing up until my miracle happened.

Then I began to wonder, "How long do I attend this meeting until I'm done? Until I graduate?" Some members dropped out after they had some time not smoking, usually a few weeks. Once, I saw a couple on the street smoking again. We spoke and one of them felt that the program didn't stick for him. I thought it was just the opposite, he didn't stick to the program.

At this writing, I've attended NicA meetings on a weekly basis for several decades, and clearly I have not graduated. I keep finding there's more to get and to give each week. The NicA principles I've practiced continue to serve me well in all of my affairs. Thank you Great Creator and my friends in recovery.

Today, I look to be grateful, rather than to graduate,
and that is a spiritual awakening.

The Twelve Steps of Nicotine Anonymous

1. We admitted we were powerless over nicotine—that our lives had become unmanageable.
2. Came to believe that a Power greater than ourselves could restore us to sanity.
3. Made a decision to turn our will and our lives over to the care of God as we understood Him.
4. Made a searching and fearless moral inventory of ourselves.
5. Admitted to God, to ourselves, and to another human being the exact nature of our wrongs.
6. Were entirely ready to have God remove all these defects of character.
7. Humbly asked Him to remove our shortcomings.
8. Made a list of all persons we had harmed, and became willing to make amends to them all.
9. Made direct amends to such people wherever possible, except when to do so would injure them or others.
10. Continued to take personal inventory and when we were wrong promptly admitted it.
11. Sought through prayer and meditation to improve our conscious contact with God as we understood Him, praying only for knowledge of His will for us and the power to carry that out.
12. Having had a spiritual awakening as the result of these steps, we tried to carry this message to nicotine users and to practice these principles in all our affairs.

The Twelve Steps reprinted and adapted with permission of Alcoholics Anonymous World Services Inc. Permission to reprint and adapt the Twelve Steps does not mean that A.A. is affiliated with this program. AA is a program of recovery from alcohol—use of the Twelve Steps in connection with programs and activities which are patterned after A.A., but which address other problems does not imply otherwise.

The Twelve Steps of Alcoholics Anonymous

1. We admitted we were powerless over alcohol—that our lives had become unmanageable. 2. Came to believe that a Power greater than ourselves could restore us to sanity. 3. Made a decision to turn our will and our lives over to the care of God as we understood Him. 4. Made a searching and fearless moral inventory of ourselves. 5. Admitted to God, to ourselves, and to another human being the exact nature of our wrongs. 6. Were entirely ready to have God remove all these defects of character. 7. Humbly asked Him to remove our shortcomings. 8. Made a list of all persons we had harmed, and became willing to make amends to them all. 9. Made direct amends to such people wherever possible, except when to do so would injure them or others. 10. Continued to take personal inventory and when we were wrong promptly admitted it.11. Sought through prayer and meditation to improve our conscious contact with God as we understood Him, praying only for knowledge of His will for us and the power to carry that out. 12. Having had a spiritual awakening as the result of these steps, we tried to carry this message to alcoholics, and practice these principles in all our affairs.

The Twelve Traditions of Nicotine Anonymous

1. Our common welfare should come first; personal recovery depends upon Nicotine Anonymous unity.
2. For our group purpose there is but one ultimate authority—a loving God as He may express Himself in our group conscience. Our leaders are but trusted servants; they do not govern.
3. The only requirement for Nicotine Anonymous membership is a desire to stop using nicotine.
4. Each group should be autonomous except in matters affecting other groups or Nicotine Anonymous as a whole.
5. Each group has but one primary purpose—to carry its message to the nicotine addict who still suffers.
6. A Nicotine Anonymous group ought never endorse, finance or lend the Nicotine Anonymous name to any related facility or outside enterprise, lest problems of money, property and prestige divert us from our primary purpose.
7. Every Nicotine Anonymous group ought to be fully self-supporting, declining outside contributions.
8. Nicotine Anonymous should remain forever non-professional, but our service centers may employ special workers.
9. Nicotine Anonymous, as such, ought never be organized; but we may create service boards or committees directly responsible to those they serve.
10. Nicotine Anonymous has no opinion on outside issues; hence the Nicotine Anonymous name ought never be drawn into public controversy.
11. Our public relations policy is based on attraction rather than promotion; we need always maintain personal anonymity at the level of press, radio, television and films.
12. Anonymity is the spiritual foundation of all our Traditions, ever reminding us to place principles before personalities.

The Twelve Traditions of A.A.

1. Our common welfare should come first: personal recovery depends upon A.A. unity. 2. For our group purpose there is but one ultimate authority—a loving God as He may express Himself in our group conscience. Our leaders are but trusted servants; they do not govern. 3. The only requirement for A.A. membership is a desire to stop drinking. 4. Each group should he autonomous except in matters affecting other groups or A.A. as a whole. 5. Each group has but one primary purpose—to carry its message to the alcoholic who still suffers. 6. An A.A. group ought never endorse. finance or lend the A.A. name to any related facility or outside enterprise lest problems of money, property and prestige divert us from our primary purpose. 7. Every A.A. group ought to be self-supporting, declining outside contributions. 8. Alcoholics Anonymous should remain forever non-professional but our service centers may employ special workers. 9. A.A.. as such. ought never he organized; but we may create service boards or committees directly responsible to those they serve. 10. Alcoholics Anonymous has no opinion on outside issues hence the A.A. name ought never he drawn into public controversy. 11. Our public relations policy is based on attraction rather than promotion; we need always maintain personal anonymity at the level of press, radio and films. 12. Anonymity is the spiritual foundation of all our traditions, ever reminding us to place principles before personalities.

INDEX

NOTES

NOTES

NOTES

NOTES